C000216383

Vita

Vital Signs

The Deadly Costs
of Health Inequality

Lee Humber

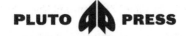

PLUTO PRESS

First published 2019 by Pluto Press
345 Archway Road, London N6 5AA

www.plutobooks.com

Copyright © Lee Humber 2019

The right of Lee Humber to be identified as the author of this work has been
asserted by him in accordance with the Copyright, Designs and Patents Act 1988.

British Library Cataloguing in Publication Data
A catalogue record for this book is available from the British Library

ISBN   978 0 7453 3834 7   Hardback
ISBN   978 0 7453 3832 3   Paperback
ISBN   978 1 7868 0424 2   PDF eBook
ISBN   978 1 7868 0426 6   Kindle eBook
ISBN   978 1 7868 0425 9   EPUB eBook

This book is printed on paper suitable for recycling and made from fully managed
and sustained forest sources. Logging, pulping and manufacturing processes are
expected to conform to the environmental standards of the country of origin.

Simultaneously printed in the United Kingdom and United States of America

Typeset by Stanford DTP Services, Northampton, England

Contents

List of Figures   vi

1   Introduction   1
2   Healthcare in the Age of Neoliberalism   12
3   Mergers, Monopolies and the 'Rising Billions'   29
4   The Social Determinants of Health   39
5   The 'Inequality Thesis'   53
6   Ageing Populations?   63
7   Health, Power and Paradigms   80
8   Legislating for Better Health?   96
9   Who's WHO?   108
10 The National Health Service: A Revolution Half Made?   119
11 Conclusion   133

Notes   136
Index   160

List of Figures

1.1   Health and care services privatised   11

2.1   Comparisons of GDP spent on healthcare   15

2.2   Global rankings of types of national health service provision   20

3.1   US life expectancies decline and fall behind OECD average   30

1

Introduction

This is a book about health. It is an analysis of what health is and what it isn't. It offers an understanding of the nature of health inequality and why it exists. Centrally, *Vital Signs* contends that health is a complex phenomenon rooted in the conditions in which we live and in history. In order, therefore, to understand and address the unequal distribution of good health and long lives which characterises the twenty-first century, we need to know about and get to grips with the significance of the periods in history when health has improved. In *Vital Signs* I ask: what is at the core of health inequality and what does history tell us we can do about it?

Vital Signs joins a growing body of work casting a critical eye on the sorts of societies that have produced the current deepening health problems. When she retired in 2017, then director general of the World Health Organisation, Dr Margaret Chan Fung Fu-chun, said: 'The challenges facing health in the 21st century are unprecedented in their complexity and universal in their impact. Under the pressures of demographic ageing, rapid urbanization, and the globalized marketing of unhealthy products, chronic non-communicable diseases have overtaken infectious diseases as the leading killers worldwide.'[1] As public health experts Anne-Emanuelle Birn and Yogan Pillay added, Dr Chan failed to touch upon the: 'preventable disease, disability, and premature death related to poor living and working conditions, limited healthcare access, discrimination, and, ultimately, the gross inequities across population groups due to highly skewed distribution of wealth, power, and resources among the world's over 7.5 billion people'.[2]

Between them Chan, Birn and Pillay clearly illustrate where the health debate and global health agenda needs to focus in the twenty-first century. In 'rapid urbanisation' Chan references not only the global spread of cities but the poor and often squalid living conditions that exist within them, affecting populations across not only the low- and middle-income countries (LMICs), but also areas and whole regions of the higher income countries (HICs), including swathes of the European Union, the US, China and Australasia. This is not simply a set of economic, social and political inequalities that exist between countries, these same inequalities in health exist within countries and within cities themselves as the work of authors such as Danny Dorling, Kate Pickett and others continues to expose. In the 'highly skewed distribution of wealth', Birn and Pillay point to the inequity and inequality that has become central to the critical analysis of global health over the last decades with a general acceptance among academics that health inequalities are linked to wealth inequality and represent a clear and present danger to the continuance of democratic societies as we have known them since the end of World War II. This same and ever-widening experience of inequality shapes the nature of disability, illness and disease such that by less than two decades into the new millennium non-communicable disease – by which Dr Chan means disease governed by the social and political environments in which we live – is the main source of premature death, shorter life expectancy and lives lived with disability. Today, the societies and environments we've built are humankind's main life-threatening enemies. To try and understand the nature of this problem and to suggest possible solutions, *Vital Signs* provides an analytical framework, based on a critical reading of health-related history and ideas. Before I do that, however, it is important to establish some broad definitions of some of the major themes, terms and institutions which will inform this critical analysis. Throughout, I refer both to broad concepts of health and to 'healthcare'. By healthcare I mean the organisation and provision of medical and social care to individuals or communities. On rare occasions in the book I focus solely on social care in order to develop analysis. The rest of the time I include health services and social care services in the term 'healthcare'.

What do we understand by the term health? Despite the fact that in many senses a biomedical understanding of health has dominated the topic, with its view of health as largely the relationship between human biology and the natural world, there is no consensus on the definitions of what health actually is, even though the concept is central not only in medicine but also in the health social sciences (e.g. medical sociology, health psychology and medical demography). This may seem strange, given the long history of medicine. Concepts of health are multidimensional and complex. For instance, Larson[3] observed that disagreements about the meaning of health are common because health is imbued with political, medical, social, economic and spiritual components. Early definitions of health focused primarily on the body's ability to function. Health was seen as a state of 'normal' function that could be disrupted by disease. An example of such a definition of health is: 'a state characterized by anatomic, physiologic, and psychological integrity; ability to perform personally valued family, work, and community roles; ability to deal with physical, biological, psychological, and social stress.'[4] Even here we see health as coterminous with what it enables us to do, and the roles it enables us to perform. Health, then, is pre-eminently a social phenomenon.

In 1948, in a radical departure from previous definitions and with the establishment of the World Health Organisation (WHO), a new definition linking health to a continual process of well-being was proposed. This definition understands health as resulting from changing relationships between 'physical, mental, and social well-being, and not merely the absence of disease and infirmity.'[5] The medical establishment, with its traditional and narrower focus on the body's relationship with disease only, remain suspicious of attempts to develop new definitions. For years following 1948, WHO's proposals were set aside as an impractical ideal.

New approaches to health began to gain purchase as late as the 1980s, with keynote documents like the Ottawa Charter of 1986 beginning to affect public and professional opinion. Following Ottawa, health began to be seen as a 'resource for living', a much more positive approach than previous absence of disease interpretations. For many, health began to be understood in a much more holistic way as 'the extent to which an individual or group is able to realize aspirations and satisfy needs and to change or cope with the environment. Health is a resource for everyday life, not the objective of living; it is a positive concept, emphasizing social and personal resources, as well as physical capacities.'[6] Aspects of health hitherto ignored were considered. Mental, intellectual, emotional and social health referred to a person's ability to handle stress, to acquire skills, to maintain relationships, all of which form resources for resiliency and independent living. In this view, health is an evolving relationship with all aspects of the environment – natural, social and political. In focusing in on the individual's – or group's – ability to 'cope with the environment' this definition highlights the impact upon us of the world in which we live. This was a clear move away from biomedical concepts of health based on individualised struggles between individual bodies and disease. Instead, health can be understood as a relational process between humans and their societies. This definition opens the door to an approach which sees health as socially determined. In order to ensure the best of health, we need to ensure the best of societies that are most supportive of the health of all. Following Ottawa, health begins to reveal itself in its true form, as an ongoing collective and political struggle against those aspects of society that threaten and undermine it.

A specifically social model of health was developed to its clearest formulation early on by the sociologist Talcott Parsons (1902–79). He defines health as 'the state of optimum capacity of an individual for the effective performance of the roles and tasks for which he has been socialized'.[7] Health in this sociological sense is more inclined towards the capacity of humans to fulfil their obligations, participate in social activities (including work) and fulfil role expectations in society in the face of structural limitations. Although 'role theory' has now largely been discredited,[8] Parsons' analysis of the sociological space for health remains important and continues to inspire others.[9]

The salutogenic health model, developed by sociologist Aaron Antonovsky, can be considered a variant of this sociologically-based approach. Salutogenesis is a term coined by Antonovsky which describes an approach focusing on factors that support human health and well-being, rather than on factors that cause disease (pathogenesis). More specifically, the 'salutogenic model' is concerned with the relationship between health, stress and coping. Antonovsky's theories reject the 'traditional medical-model dichotomy separating health and illness'. Instead he describes the relationship as a continuous variable, what he called the 'health-ease versus dis-ease continuum'.[10] The work of French philosopher Georges Canguilhem is another insightful approach, offering a historically based analysis of the relationship between 'normal' and ill health. His brilliant critique, 'The Normal and the Pathological', shows that a fixed state of something called 'normal' health is not possible and that the concept normal itself is a relational process, an idea taken up more broadly in sociology. Canguilhem demonstrates how the ideas of the normal and the pathological, far from being scientifically determined and static, are value concepts shaped by political, economic and techno-logical values linked to institutional power: 'A norm draws its meaning, function and value from the fact of the existence, outside itself, of what does not meet the requirement it serves. The normal is not a static or peaceful, but dynamic and polemical concept.'[11] For Canguilhem, the concept of 'normal' – including the idea of 'normal' health – serves specific ideological and political functions at specific points in history. His insights continue to provide a basis for critiquing the biomedical assumptions and methodologies that continue to dominate how we view health.

Before we look in more detail at the health inequality academic literature it is worth sketching out some of the major developments at the institutional, policy and programme levels that have influenced health inequality. WHO, a specialised agency of the United Nations specifically concerned with public health, came into being in 1948. It is responsi-ble for key publications like the *World Health Report* and the worldwide *Health Survey*, and World Health Day. Historically, its roots are in the sanitation movements of the mid-nineteenth century. Between 1851 and 1938 a series of International Sanitary Conferences worked to combat diseases such as yellow fever and bubonic plague. The movement's major success came following the conference of 1892 when measures to combat 'King Cholera', the nineteenth century's most lethal infectious disease, were internationally recognised. Taking its modern form in 1948, WHO has been involved with numerous health initiatives including those against smallpox in the 1960s and HIV/AIDS in the 1980s. Its core objectives include such functions as acting as the directing and coordinating body for international health work, and establishing and maintaining effective collaboration with the United Nations, specialised agencies, governmental health administrations, professional groups and other organisations. Since the beginning of our current century a key growth area for the organisation in regard to collaborations has been via so-called public–private partnerships (PPP), a topic discussed in detail in Chapter 9. Keynote documents, programmes and declarations of intent that WHO has spearheaded include the Jakarta Declaration of 1997, the Bangkok Charter of 2005 and before those, the Ottawa Charter for Health Promotion of 1986, which established five key areas for health promotion that are still largely dominant today. These include building healthy public policy, creating supportive environments, strengthening community action, developing personal skills and reorienting healthcare services towards prevention of illness and promotion of health. As this shows, WHO's role centres on initiating and collecting research and finding ways of putting findings into action.

Preceding the Ottawa Charter was the Alma-Ata Declaration, passed at the International Conference on Primary Health Care held in Kazakhstan in 1978. It expressed the need for urgent action by all governments, all health and development workers, and the world community in developing primary healthcare to protect and promote the health of all people. It was the first international declaration underlining the importance of primary healthcare. Primary healthcare includes that provided in communities as a first port of call through doctors, community clinics and so on. The centrality of the primary healthcare approach has since been accepted in principle by member countries of WHO. The Alma-Ata Declaration is a major milestone in the field of public health, identifying primary healthcare as the key area in pursuit of the global goal of 'Health for All'.

WHO has two main sources of funding. First, its member states pay assessed contributions (calculated relative to a country's wealth and population), which, since 2006, make up around 25 per cent of WHO's revenues.[12] The rest comes from voluntary contributions. For the two-year budget period 2010–11, 53 per cent of the voluntary contributions came directly from governments that for various reasons chose to go beyond their annual dues; 21 per cent came from other UN bodies (such as UNICEF, UNDP and UNAIDS) and other multilateral bodies (such as the Global Alliance for Vaccines and Immunization); and 18 per cent came from philanthropic foundations, such as the Bill & Melinda Gates Foundation (BMGF), the UN Foundation and the Rockefeller Foundation. It has been argued that partnerships with so-called 'philanthrocapitalism' like BMGF and the Rockefeller Foundation, along with relationships with 'big pharma' via the Global Alliance for Vaccines, leave WHO open to manipulation by private for-profit interests, an accusation that WHO strenuously denies.[13] There can be little doubt, however, that the increasing influence of private companies via the extension of PPP relationships has impacted upon WHO's role. Working with any partner, including private business, necessarily means compromise, as I show below.

The Health Inequality Literature

In a paper published in 2015, Kate Pickett and Richard Wilkinson identified in excess of 140 research papers published over the recent past detailing the many and varied relationships between wealth inequality and health. As the authors say, 'The body of evidence strongly suggests that income inequality affects population health and wellbeing ... large income differences have damaging health and social consequences ... and in most countries inequality is increasing'.[14] Pickett and Wilkinson have been at the centre of this field of study since the publication of their groundbreaking study, *The Spirit Level: Why More Equal Societies Almost Always Do Better*,[15] in 2009. In brief, the book argues that inequality, and in particular income inequality, impacts on the health of whole populations, 'eroding trust, increasing anxiety and illness, [and] encouraging excessive consumption'. For the authors inequality is bad for everyone, not just those at the poorer end of the income continuum. It claims that across a range of different health and social problems including physical and mental health, drug abuse, education, imprisonment, obesity, social mobility, trust and community life, violence, teenage pregnancies and child well-being, outcomes are significantly worse in more unequal countries. The bigger the wealth gap, the worse the average health of the whole population, not just the poor. The book sold hundreds of thousands of copies globally, being translated into dozens of languages. Their follow-up book, *The Inner Level*, published in 2018, looks at the more personal, individual effects of inequality.[16] As Wilkinson says of the book:

> It takes a whole argument and evidence about the effects of inequality to a deeper and more intimate level. In 'The Spirit Level' we were dealing with things about society 'out there' – the size of the prison population, homicide rates, obesity rates and so on. But this takes it into the sphere of our social fears and anxieties ... Worries about self-worth: all the things that make social contact sometimes seem rather awkward and stressful.[17]

In large part underpinning the approach taken by these authors is the pioneering and continuing work and influence of Michael Marmot. Marmot has become one of the lynchpins in the global health debates around inequality. Currently director of the University College London Institute of Health Equity, as well as a range of other influential roles, Marmot has led research groups on health inequalities for over 35 years. He was chair of the Commission on Social Determinants of Health (CSDH), which was set up by the World Health Organization in 2005, and produced 'Closing the Gap in a Generation'[18] in August 2008 which I analyse in Chapters 4 and 9. He leads the English Longitudinal Study of Ageing, and is engaged in several international research efforts on the social determinants of health. He served as president of the British Medical Association (BMA) from 2010 to 2011. In the UK one of the most influential studies in which he was involved was the series of 'Whitehall Studies' of British civil servants, focusing on heart and other disease patterns.[19] Phase one of the Whitehall Study examined over 18,000 male civil servants between the ages of 20 and 64, and was conducted over a period of ten years, beginning in 1967. A second phase was conducted from 1985 to 1988 and examined the health of 10,308 civil servants aged 35 to 55, of whom two-thirds were men and one-third women.[20]

The studies found a strong association between grade levels of civil servant employment and mortality rates from a range of causes: the lower the grade, the higher the mortality rate. Men in the lowest grade (messengers, doorkeepers, etc.) had a mortality rate three times higher than that of men in the highest grade (administrators). This effect has since been observed in other studies and named the 'status syndrome'.[21] For Marmot and his co-researchers, autonomy, a sense of control over your life and social connectedness – the supporting social networks on which individuals can draw, rather than financial resources, living and employment conditions or access to medical services, have the greatest impact on your health and life expectancy. Marmot went on to develop this idea further in his book, *Status Syndrome*, published in 2006. As Marmot writes: 'The lower in hierarchy you are, the less likely it is that you will have full control over your life and opportunities for full social participation ... Autonomy and social participation are so important for health that their lack leads to deterioration in health.'[22] This idea – that the key influence on the differing health expectations of a population are to do with social status – is a dominant one in the inequality literature and one I critique in detail in Chapter 5.

The social geographer Danny Dorling's body of work is extensive, impressive and highly influential, particularly (but not only) with regard to health inequality in the UK. Dorling has been writing on inequalities since the mid-1990s and has established himself as a major commentator on a wide range of topics, from health inequality to social justice more generally. His 2018 book, *Peak Inequality: Britain's Ticking Time Bomb*,[23] explores how health inequality fits into wider political debates ranging from those concerned with the condition and future of education and education systems in the UK and beyond, to the Brexit saga in the UK between 2018 and 2019. The final section of his book, 'Future', reads like a manifesto for an incoming reformist party, offering a wide range of stimulating ideas ending with the paper, 'Why Corbyn's Moral Clarity Could Propel Him to Number 10'.[24]

Writing with Kate Pickett, Dorling provides a very useful critique of *Fair Society, Healthy Lives: Strategic Review of Health Inequalities in England*, better known as 'The Marmot Review', published in 2010.[25] Like other enquiries into UK health and health inequalities the report was commissioned by one political party in power and came to publication as another took over. *The Black Report*,[26] for example, was similarly commissioned by a Labour government and came to publication under a Conservative one. As Dorling and Pickett point out, this has meant that very few of the recommendations made by the report have been enacted. There is a political problem with *Fair Society* then. As the authors point out, there are methodological problems too. For example, Dorling and Pickett argue that the report fails to address inequalities at 'the top end of the social hierarchy, as well as at the bottom … there is no suggestion that a maximum income or a constraint on the ratio of top-to-bottom incomes' should be made and acted upon.[27] Comparison is made between the recommendations made in *Fair Society* and those made by the *Black Report*, nearly 40 years previously. Ideas in *Fair Society* like 'Give every child the best start in life' and 'Create fair employment and good work for all' are, the authors believe, 'unlikely to scare the horses'[28] in government. Compare that to recommendation seven, for example, of the *Black Report* which details: 'We recommend that school health statistics should routinely provide, in relation to occupational class, the results of tests of hearing, vision and measures of height and weight. As a first step we recommend that local health authorities, in consultation with educational authorities, select a representative sample of schools in which assessments on a routine basis be initiated.'[29] The *Black Report* is a micro analysis and set of practical and practicable suggestions based on a class analysis of health inequalities, while for Dorling and Pickett, Marmot's review is not.

In an earlier work, *Unequal Health*, Dorling focuses on some of the more conceptual issues surrounding the health inequality debate, in the process mounting a somewhat hesitant defence of the so-called 'inequality thesis' pioneered by Wilkinson and Pickett:

> Grand theories such as the inequality thesis are currently out of vogue in an academia where the fashion of the day is to say everything is all very complicated and contingent. Grand theories are, by their nature, unlikely to be true. That is because they tend to contradict each other so only a few can hold water … However, a grand theory may be proposed that turns out largely to appear to hold water.[30]

I look in detail at the inequality thesis in Chapter 5.

The predominant feature of debate about health and healthcare services globally over the course of the twenty-first century is the increasing privatisation of provision, with services previously run as a public good by the governments of nation states being taken over, wholesale or in parts, by private healthcare providers. Chapter 2 uses the case study of developments in the UK to discuss this at length, but this tendency is far from a UK issue only. Privatisation in its various guises is 'spreading across Europe's health services like a rash', writes John Lister of Keep Our NHS Public and Health Campaigns Together (see Figure 1.1). EU member states' health systems are split between those based on employment-related health insurance and those financed centrally via general taxation. Both have been subject to political and policy pressures, including from EU-level, supportive of a growing role for private sector companies in this traditionally public service.[31]

Vital Signs is organised into two halves. The first half explores the nature of the health problem, looking at the current dominant paradigm in healthcare and with regard to health philosophies today, one based on the idea that healthcare and health generally are commodities to be bought and sold on a market in health. Chapters 2 and 3 examine how this paradigm is being and has been established, using the UK and the US healthcare systems as case studies. Chapters 4 and 5 compare and contrast two ways of understanding health problems currently. The first is a social determinant approach to health which points to how

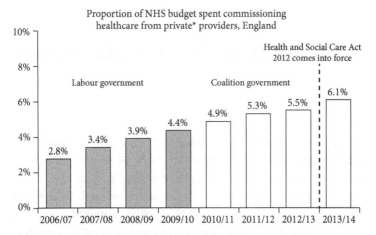

* Excludes local government, charities and the voluntary sector

Figure 1.1   Health and care services privatised

Source: Department for Health 9response to Full Fact query)

health-governing social and political issues such as housing, diet and employment impact on our health. The second and related approach is encapsulated by the so-called inequality thesis, which regards understanding the nature and impact of health inequality as the key element to grasp in order to effect change.

Chapter 7 is, in many ways, a pivotal chapter. In it I explain Thomas Kuhn's concept of dominant paradigms and paradigm shifts and how this concept can begin to help us understand how health is governed and can change. I do this by looking at the health paradigm shifts implicit in three of the key socio-political events of the modern era, the English, French and Russian revolutions.

This brings us to the second half of the book, which looks at ways of addressing health inequality. I discuss, at length, historically important phases of when health and healthcare systems improved. I interrogate the role of such international bodies as WHO and others, and investigate the record of governments in the reformist tradition in protecting and improving our health. For example, Chapter 10 looks in detail at the historical roots of the National Health Service (NHS) and asks, was the NHS in fact a revolution half made?

2

Healthcare in the Age of Neoliberalism

London, 15 November 2017: Research linking cuts in government health spending to higher mortality rates in England has been published today in the BMJ Open. Leading medical researchers from universities including Oxford, Cambridge, and UCL found that spending cuts, in particular cuts to public expenditure on social care, are associated with an increased number of deaths in patients over 60. The study is the first of its kind to link the impact of health and social care funding gaps on the population. The research found that spending constraints between 2010 [and] 2014 were associated with an estimated 45,368 more deaths than anticipated compared to pre-2010 trends, with nearly 120,000 excess deaths estimated between 2010 and 2017. Moving forward, mortality projections indicate up to 100 excess deaths per day, unless action is taken. Deaths were predominantly in care home and homecare residents, with NHS hospitals performing better than expected in the 2010–2014 period.[1]

Neoliberalism kills. During the twenty-first century, as part of an economic and political era stretching back to the late 1970s, the world and everything in it has been characterised by what has become known as neoliberalism. Healthcare, and as I show throughout health itself, along with ways of conceptualising health, are no exception to this. Healthcare models globally have fundamentally changed over the last half century and they continue to do so. Previously, in the years following World War II, governments were primarily responsible for attending to the health needs of their populations, developing versions of state-driven welfare provision to provide medical and social care directly. From the late 1970s onwards this began to change, and increasingly healthcare came to be dominated by private healthcare capital, touching every corner of the globe. From the UK to Tajikistan private healthcare has come to dominate large sectors of health and social care provision.

Today, in the UK the 'independent sector' provides nearly 90 per cent of all care services; in the remote region of Badakhshan in Tajikistan the Aga Khan Foundation, along with other multilateral organisations and non-governmental organisations, has created a 'sustainable market'[2] in healthcare commodities following the decline of Russian influence in the region. As Chapter 3 discusses in detail, what has become known as a medical–industrial complex, comprising vast multinational companies many of which are based in the US, has spread its reach over the past 50 years. In the process, an idea has taken root that it is perfectly legitimate that we should regard healthcare – and indeed health itself – as a commodity, something to be bought and sold on a neoliberal market controlled by private industry seeking to generate profit.

How should we understand neoliberalism? At a conceptual level, neoliberalism is characterised by an emphasis on economies operating on the basis of market principles, that is by allowing capitalists in small firms to big business to compete against each other without being restricted by the interventions of government through industrial legislation, corporate tax and so on. In practice, of course, the reality is very different and governments constantly intervene to support and rescue failing firms and whole industries. The most obvious example as I write is the practice of 'quantitative easing' introduced following the global financial crash of 2008. Through it, governments for the past ten years have provided cheap credit in order to provide vital support for industries otherwise likely to go under. Neoliberalism infers low corporate and personal tax, favouring the wealthy, the flexible use of labour which has contextualised short-term and zero hour contracts along with a decline in the rights of trade unionists, and a belief that the capitalist market is the engine of growth for life improvement – and better health – generally. Neoliberalism assumes various forms around the world, and I analyse these in health contexts, exploring the nature of the medical–industrial complex, how its institutionalisation of the idea of health as a commodity impacts upon national healthcare arrangements and the nature of the PPPs established between bodies such as WHO and the so-called philanthrocapitalism of the BMGF and other independent sector bodies. But first, let us begin with an in-depth analysis of how this process of the commodification of health has developed, and continues to develop, in the UK.

In the UK, since before the beginning of the twenty-first century, the growth of neoliberalism in the healthcare sector has been actively encouraged and facilitated by successive governments of all parties. Especially since 2010, but also in evidence before that, a flood of legislation seeking to reconfigure healthcare systems has changed the face of services. Most recently, two Health and Social Care Acts (2012/2015), a Care Act (2014), the Five Year Forward View (2014), 'vanguards', 'Multispecialty Community Providers' (MCPs) and the 'Primary and Acute Care System' (PACS) all passed into law between 2010 and 2018 and had major impacts on healthcare at governance, systemic and service level. Arguments governments have used to open up formerly state-run services to the private sector include the idea that given rising demand for health services, an ageing population and improved medication along with the growth of health-related technology, both of which help people live longer, governments can no longer afford to maintain a nationalised healthcare service. In the process, over the past two decades the NHS has variously been accused of being 'too big', too expensive, inefficient and bureaucratic. As a result, it has been argued, governments need the help of private business, set free by the tenets of neoliberalism, allowing private capital to intervene to develop profit-generating care provision to fill the gaps left by this decrepit and outmoded welfare approach to healthcare. As a result, since before the 1990s private capital has made huge inroads into healthcare services.

One very obvious consequence of this is that in care services throughout Europe neoliberal, profit-driven approaches have pushed services to near crisis point. In the UK, 47 major care providers closed in 2014–15 alone and this trend is likely to have accelerated since then.[3] In 2017 in Oxfordshire during the first part of 2017 four or five providers went out of business each month, causing a crisis that saw council administration staff being sent into residential homes to provide care themselves.[4] Across Europe, state-run healthcare provision of all kinds is under intense pressure as a result of years of government-led austerity contextualised by the for-profit approach of neoliberal healthcare, with – especially but not only in Spain, Portugal, Ireland and Greece – the selling off and slashed funding of publicly run healthcare provision.[5] As I show in Chapter 3, the situation in the 'market leader' in commodified health, the US, is worse and continues to deteriorate.

This global crisis presents complex problems for employers and governments. Healthcare services are an essential part of how countries manage and maintain their working populations. Since at least what the Marxist historian Eric Hobsbawm calls the 'second industrial revolution'[6] in the second half of the nineteenth century, governments worldwide have accepted the necessity of intervening in some way to support a population's health and social welfare, in order to ensure an adequately healthy workforce. Since that time governments, at least in the Highly Industrialised Countries, have conceded the need to commit resources in order to do so, the amount being determined by historically specific combinations of social and political forces. The problem for governments and employers is how to ensure that healthcare services are robust enough to guarantee a healthy workforce while at the same time sticking to neoliberal agendas including reining in state expenditure. To explore the complexity of the relationships between governments and private healthcare the following is an analysis of primary and secondary healthcare developments in the UK.

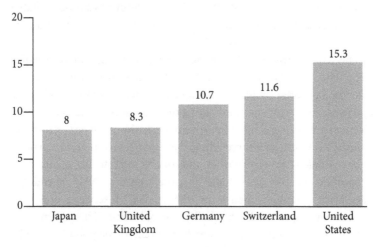

Figure 2.1   Comparisons of GDP spent on healthcare

In the UK, spending on healthcare as a percentage of gross domestic product (GDP) is around the average for EU countries generally at around 8.3 per cent (see Figure 2.1).[7] For 2017–18, planned spending for the Department of Health in England was approximately £124.7 billion. Though funding for the Department of Health grew, the rate of growth slowed considerably compared to historical trends. The Department of Health budget will have grown by 1.2 per cent in real terms between 2009–10 and 2020–1. This is far below the long-term average increases in health spending of approximately 4 per cent a year (above inflation) since the NHS was established in 1948.[8] In 2018, it was below the rate of increase needed to maintain current standards of service based on projections by the Office of Budget Responsibility (4.3 per cent a year).[9] In 2017, the government provided an additional £2.8 billion for day-to-day spending on staff salaries and medicines, partly in response to the chronic shortages of staff which persist. Further funding on top of this amount was promised for future pay awards for NHS staff such as nurses, midwives and paramedics. The government committed to an extra £10 billion in capital funding over the parliament for investment in buildings, facilities and equipment. Central government committed to £4 billion of this amount with the remainder coming from private financing and sales of surplus NHS land and assets, along with some private finance through PPPs. By the end of 2018, this had already been shown to be highly risky with the collapse of the giant Carillion building company which had been awarded several giant NHS-related building contracts, leaving numerous projects incomplete.[10]

The 2018 British Social Attitudes survey shows that in 1997 half of the public were dissatisfied with the NHS. Between 2001 and 2010 satisfaction increased significantly as a result of increases in NHS funding and consequent reductions in waiting times for accident and emergency, elective treatment and other improvements in the quality of patient care. British Social Attitudes surveys have consistently shown health spending to be one of the top two priorities, and surveys indicate that an increasing proportion of the population support boosting NHS spending.[11] Healthcare spending impacts on the quality of services, and more fundamentally potentially the quality of people's lives. This presents governments attempting to move away from a reliance on publicly provided services to private healthcare with major political problems.

The NHS employs over 1.5 million people, representing the fifth biggest single employer in the world.[12] It has consistently been accused of being unwieldy, inefficient and bureaucratic. However, a 2017 review by the Office for Budgetary Responsibility estimates that productivity in the healthcare sector grows by 1.2 per cent a year, indicating that the NHS is producing more (i.e. hospital activity) for the resources it is given. This growth in NHS productivity is lower than the 2.2 per cent long-term growth in the productivity of the wider economy over the past 40 years, and studies show the NHS has maintained its productivity growth since the 2008/9 recession even as whole economy productivity has stagnated.[13] Healthcare is labour-intensive and heavily based on human interaction and customised care. As such, efficiency improvements through the use of technologies and automation, the trend in all other industries, is much more difficult. Despite this, the healthcare industry continues to gamble vast sums of money and its hopes for future global profit on medical technological developments.

As the Kings Fund argues, lower healthcare productivity growth in the long run is to be expected, with its focus on outcomes like additional years of healthy life and well-being. But we should ask a more funda- mental question of this concept of healthcare productivity: is it possible even to apply it with regard to health? Certainly, in terms of ratios of nurses to patients in hospitals the numbers have fallen, with the safety limit of one nurse for every seven patients set by National Institute for Health and Care Excellence guidelines in 2018 regularly exceeded.[14] Reducing staff numbers and making the rest work harder (increasing the rate of exploitation) is a tried and tested way in which industrial capitalism has traditionally sought to generate more profit, and this is evidenced in healthcare generally through a wealth of recent research. At a European-wide level, Rachel Tansey of the Corporate Europe Observa- tory reports that squeezing profits for shareholders out of health services contextualises deteriorating working conditions across the EU. Worse pay, reduced staff levels, greater workloads and more stress all negatively affect safety and quality of care. Greater health inequality is fostered as private, for-profit providers 'cherry pick' lower-risk and paying patients, while higher-risk and poorer patients, or those needing emergency care, remain reliant on under-resourced (thanks to austerity) public health service provision. A combined set of EU-level pressures have helped create a pro-privatisation environment. While there is no single channel of influence in Brussels of private healthcare interests (e.g. private hospitals, private health insurance, etc.), there is evidence of corporate lobbying influenced by big business groups, companies and think tanks.[15] This, and a shared underpinning ideology centred on the idea that health markets are better at providing for our health needs, helps feed the financial and political agenda that encourages more privatised models of healthcare. The model rests on the view of healthcare as a commodity, bought and sold on a healthcare market. Moreover, health itself becomes a commodity, secured and maintained by an individual's ability to afford sufficient health-promoting goods. As Thomas Kuhn would put it, this market-oriented view of health forms the 'dominant paradigm' in health and healthcare today.[16]

In the NHS, nurses' productivity has increased. However, and much more importantly, we can only continue with an assessment of productivity measured by 'additional years of healthy life', as the Kings Fund and other health political economists would like us to, if we continue with what is the complete myth that healthcare is solely – or even primarily – the key determining factor of a populations' health. As I show in Chapter 4, developing an approach pioneered by WHO, health is fundamentally determined by a wide range of far more general social factors over which healthcare workers can have no control. As such, it is simply not possible to attempt to measure the productivity of healthcare workers as political economists would like to. Care, and the outcomes of care, are not commodities produced and for sale in the same way that a shirt or a car is. Health is far more complex than that.

Is the NHS bureaucratic? Since the Health and Social Care Act 2012, many new organisations have entered the NHS. There are now more than 200 clinical commissioning groups (CCGs) that purchase hospital, ambulance, community and mental health services. Health and well-being boards, clinical senates, academic health science networks and sustainability and transformation plans have been introduced. The growth in the number of different organisations, and the pre-existing separation between organisations that purchase and provide NHS healthcare, significantly increase the costs of delivering healthcare, as well as adding significantly to bureaucracies. Frontline NHS organisations are overseen by different national bodies, such as the Care Quality Commission, which regulates care quality; NHS Improvement, which regulates NHS providers; and NHS England, which oversees CCGs. The CCG model itself has been variously criticised as problematic in the UK context.[17] The cost of nationally mandated data collection requests from these bodies may be as much as £300–£500 million a year.[18] The additional bureaucracy is a direct result of the initiatives to turn the NHS into a profit-generating, market-driven enterprise. A state-run NHS was and remains a complex bureaucracy but no more so than any other major industrial employer. Despite staff shortages, ward closures and a decline in public spending, the overall efficiency and huge popularity of the state-run NHS model remains, and compares very favourably with other European models and those elsewhere in the world. As Figure 2.2 shows, the NHS comes first in a range of categories measuring aspects of standards of care when compared with eleven other highly industrialised countries.

At primary care level, systemic and ideological changes associated with neoliberalism impact on a daily basis on general practice as the traditional roles of community doctors are reconfigured by the increasing commodification of health. General practitioners (GPs) are required to establish the ethnic and religious backgrounds of their patients as a way of rationing health provision through their responsibility to follow GMS1 Form and Prevent strategy duties. Meanwhile, in hospitals by 2018 it was becoming increasingly common for patients from black, Asian and minority ethnic backgrounds to be asked for documentary evidence of their rights to treatment.[19] Through the business-oriented auspices of CCGs, with responsibilities to decide on health priorities in specific regions, local GP surgeries have become semi-independent businesses themselves, with a responsibility to run surgeries to strictly controlled budgets. This has put additional pressure on GPs, who are not trained as business managers. As a result, in many areas 'super-partnerships' have evolved, bringing together surgeries to produce fewer, centralised facilities in order to generate sufficient economies of scale to support the employment of business management specialists. More business managers and fewer doctors, with surgeries run at low staff levels with the increased use of locums, have resulted. Research suggests that this is already beginning to erode surgery–community links.[20] Big pharma, the network of multinational drugs companies, impact upon drug provision agendas such that GPs are constrained with regard to prescribing over-the-counter drugs.[21] Primary care in the UK is becoming focused on fewer, bigger, more impersonal GP surgeries, run primarily with tight budgets in mind, given more policing roles and subject to an ever more powerful global medical–industrial complex.

'Super-partnerships' are indicative of a much broader trend occurring in the UK and beyond, a trend that since the 1990s has already reshaped social care and which continues to influence healthcare generally. Since the early 1990s, an accelerating process of what is known as the

	AUS	CAN	FRA	GER	NETH	NZ	NOR	SWE	SWIZ	UK	US
Overall Ranking (2013)	4	10	9	5	5	7	7	3	2	1	11
Quality Care	2	9	8	7	5	4	11	10	3	1	5
Effective Care	4	7	9	6	5	2	11	10	8	1	3
Safe Care	3	10	2	6	7	9	11	5	4	1	7
Coordinated Care	4	8	9	10	5	2	7	11	3	1	6
Patient-Centred Care	5	8	10	7	3	6	11	9	2	1	4
Access	8	9	11	2	4	7	6	4	2	1	9
Cost-Related Problem	9	5	10	4	8	6	3	1	7	1	11
Timeliness of Care	6	11	10	4	2	7	8	9	1	3	5
Efficiency	4	10	8	9	7	3	4	2	6	1	11
Equity	5	9	7	4	8	10	6	1	2	2	11
Healthy Lives	4	8	1	7	5	9	6	2	3	10	11
Health Expenditures/Capita, 2011**	$3,800	$4,522	$4,118	$4,495	$5,099	$3,182	$5,669	$3,925	$5,643	$3,405	$8,508

Country Rankings   Top 2*   Middle   Bottom 2*

Notes: * Includes ties. ** Expenditures shown in $US PPP (purchasing power parity); Australian $ are from 2010.

Source: Calculated by The Commonwealth Fund based on 2011 International Health Policy Survey of Sicker Adults; 2012 International Health Policy Survey of Primary Care Physicians; 2013 International Health Policy Survey; Commonwealth Fund *National Scorecard 2011*; World Health Organization and Organization for Economic Cooperation and Development, *OECD Health Data, 2013* (Paris: OECD, Nov. 2013).

Figure 2.2   Global rankings of types of national health service provision

centralisation of capital has set the context of the development of the UK's care sector. This is not just a UK phenomenon. Globally, there has been a fundamental shift in resources away from the public sector towards independent providers.

In 1993, the independent sector in the UK, comprising charities, not-for-profit voluntary and for-profit agencies, provided just 5 per cent of care services. By 2013, this had risen to 89 per cent.[22] There are over 160,000 charities and 70,000 social enterprises overall, with a combined annual income greater than £60 billion, employing 1.6 million workers in 2012. This represents over 4 per cent of UK GDP and 5 per cent of UK employment. It is a huge and increasingly important employment and economic part of modern societies.

In the UK, since the 1980s, governments have worked hard to create this privatised and semi-privatised independent sector industry in social care, initially seeking to concentrate financial resources – through local government grants and loans – in the hands of a plethora of relatively small, independent sector businesses. As the *Financial Times* pointed out, over time this strategy changed so that rather than enabling a further extensive growth of small care providers, governments aimed to concentrate services in fewer, bigger organisations: 'Further promotion by the government of alternative models used by the private sector, combined with the removal of barriers to the sector's increasing participation, will create a positive environment for ongoing consolidation and Mergers and Acquisitions across healthcare services.'[23]

By far the largest spend for local authorities funding social care provision are services for older people and for people with learning disabilities. For example, in Oxfordshire these services account for nearly 70 per cent of the total spend, and this is representative of national trends.[24] In terms of provision for people with learning disabilities, business analysts LaingBuisson show that the total value of the UK's combined market for residential and non-residential care was £8.2 billion in 2012–13.[25] Contracting out services remains a key strategy for local government, representing a huge saving for local authorities who continue to suffer from and implement welfare spending cuts. Between 2013 and 2018, central government welfare funding fell by a massive £5 billion,[26] partially explaining the continued movement of social care provision to the much cheaper independent sector. Financial constraints mean local governments use the independent sector based very largely on cost, regardless of questions of quality of service.

Though local authority contracts and funding remain central to financing independent sector social care provision since 2010 in particular, the sector has been strongly encouraged to take on debt to finance care. Social Impact Investment (SII) schemes have been made available to independent sector organisations by governments to wean them off a reliance on public sector funding. SII schemes are a way for governments to provide incentives, in the form of tax relief and other benefits, to support individual and corporate investors to provide cheap loans to social care agencies.[27] Between 2000 and 2014, there were 25 SIIs, including Bridges Ventures (owned by Sir Ronald Cohen, 'the father of British venture capital' and 'the father of social investment'), Futurebuilders, Big Society Capital and others.[28] Funds were primarily provided for fixed capital purposes to support the independent sector to build homes and capacity generally. All of the SIIs encourage private and multinational investors who require a return on their investment, even the relatively low one agreed by the nature of the SII schemes. Services are provided by a complex system of 'demand' organisations and agencies (which include cooperatives, charities, social enterprises, mainstream businesses and government commissioning) which are serviced by a range of 'supply' agencies via another range of 'intermediary' organisations. Supply agencies include individual investors, institutional investors, government investment, charitable foundations, philanthropists and corporates. The intermediaries include social banks, fund managers, infrastructural elements, instruments (or investment schemes) and Community Development Finance Institutions.[29] This complex, three-tier system has evolved to replace the central government-local authority-service provision relationship of pre-1980s welfarism. As yet, little research has been published showing how much money is absorbed at each stage of this new system of what has been termed 'philanthrocapitalism' through staffing, administration and other leakage, but it is likely that resources that should have gone to care are substantially reduced in this way.[30] As with the complex bureaucracies implicit in broader changes in the NHS discussed above, the market in social care has not made things less bureaucratic and inefficient but more so.

The UK care sector has seen an influx of international capital. Anchorage Capital, better known for its purchase of MGM Studios, is one of the more prominent corporations to buy into the UK residential care industry (or rather in its real estate – most often these companies have little interest in care).[31] Multinational corporations lease land and properties back to care organisations who are then required to pay rent with resources that would otherwise go to provide care for service users. Accountancy firm Moore Stephens reported recently: 'Many care homes have ... lost control over their increasing property costs by selling ownership of the property they occupy to an investor and then renting the property back from the same investor with pre-agreed rent increases they can no longer afford'.[32]

Health Care American (HCA) is a huge US healthcare conglomerate, with a market capitation of over $28 billion. It is another big fish in the UK healthcare's pond. It has formed HCA NHS Ventures as an investment arm in charge of UK interventions. It has built several state of the art cancer facilities such as the Harley Street Clinic at University College Hospital offering, its advertising literature says, cancer care with 'stunning panoramic views across London'.[33]

It is apparent that the very idea of financing care services through encouraging relatively small, independent sector organisations to take on debt is problematic. A range of consequences have been identified, including the problems that independent sector agencies face in generating profits to repay loans. Evidence suggests that funding services through loans also drives organisations away from the core purpose of their services, in search of profits to finance repayment often resulting in staff and service cuts.[34]

Debt levels in the UK residential care sector have been perilously high since the financial crash of 2008. Research in 2013 found over 700 companies were 'zombie' businesses with debts higher than assets.[35] This was during a period of historically low interest rates since 2010. Even a small rise in rates, the mere threat of which in 2018 sent share prices tumbling,[36] would have disastrous consequences in this already extremely fragile environment. Shares in market leaders like Four Seasons, Care UK and NHP in 2018 were widely regarded as junk bonds, or sub-investment status, and dangerously risky for investors to buy.[37] NHP, for example, had debts of £1.8 billion in 2013. In December 2016, the *Financial Times* reported that Four Seasons had closed or sold 51 homes for older people during 2016, seeking to cut costs. It was due to dispose of a similar number in 2017–18 contextualising the return of fewer, bigger institutions.[38] Nearly a quarter of independent sector care providers were likely to 'exit the market' in 2018 as a result of debt and lack of central and local government support, causing a 'loss of 40,000 beds in the independent social care market, and the worsening of a bed-blocking crisis already in evidence across much of the NHS'.[39] A report by the GMB, a leading union for care industry workers, showed that one way ailing care homes are attempting to deal with this is by taking on more fee-paying customers, with private residents paying on average 40 per cent more than publicly funded residents.[40] LaingBuisson reports that 2015 saw the first fall in the number of places in residential homes for a decade, with 3,000 fewer beds available.[41] More debt, fewer beds and a two-tier system in social care are some of the consequences of this expanding market in healthcare provision, underpinning health inequalities and the growing social divide in health outcomes across the UK and populations elsewhere.

The shortage of available beds in the care sector has a knock-on effect in hospitals which are increasingly forced to retain patients who would otherwise be discharged. This so-called 'bed-blocking' crisis is an expression of the broader problems in the social care sector, and a direct consequence of the marketisation of services. Buyouts, bond issues, refinancing and other corporate and ownership strategies make the residential care sector very difficult for local authorities to monitor or control, even if they wanted to.[42] Left to the anarchy of the market, with no central body overseeing and planning provision, with a plethora of independent sector organisations competing for scarce resources and needing to make a profit from them, with their buildings rented from multinational corporate conglomerates beyond the reach of local control, the system bumps along in crisis mode and will continue to do so until radical solutions are found.

This has been shown to be impacting upon mortality rates already, with research linking cuts in government health spending to higher mortality rates in England published in the *BMJ* in 2015. Leading medical researchers from universities including Oxford, Cambridge and UCL found that spending cuts, in particular cuts to public expenditure on social care, are associated with an increased number of deaths in patients over 60.[43]

Great hope is placed by the medical industry in technological advance. Technology includes anything from ways of using e-technology to the development of new drugs and medical procedures. The west London borough of Fulham was one of the first to offer online consultations with doctors via laptops and mobile phone apps. Southwark Council in south London have moved to the extensive use of motion detectors in the homes of those the council cares for. Jay Stickland, director of Southwark Council's adult social care department in 2018, extols the virtues of motion detectors and other technologies to replace care workers in older people's homes and elsewhere: 'We could pop in [to see someone] at lunchtime, at one o'clock. [But at] five past one, she could be on the floor. So, there's no real value to this.'[44] Motion detector systems of monitoring, online doctor's appointments and other e-technology means healthcare becomes much more flexible and a potentially cheaper commodity for those in control of it. However, research suggests that the quality of care resulting from the decline in human contact inferred by these developments is likely to fall.[45]

The increasing use and misuse of medication is a trend widely recognised as a major problem in care homes in both the UK, the US and elsewhere. For example, research commissioned by NHS England in July 2015 found that:

There is a much higher rate of prescribing of medicines associated with mental illness amongst people with learning disabilities than the general population, often more than one medicine in the same class, and in the majority of cases with no clear justification; Medicines are often used for long periods without adequate review; There is poor communication with parents and carers, and between different healthcare providers.[46]

The increasing use of sedation for older people, those with a learning disability and other vulnerable groups is a consequence and explanation of declining numbers of staff, as well as being, for the employers, a cheaper alternative. Joe Greener points out that the marketisation of care provision has seen the quality of service deteriorate consistently over the past 20 years.[47] Staff cuts mean the work for those left is 'highly routinised within a system of bureaucratic control which emphasises the physical, "dirty" tasks of care'. Fewer overcrowded homes, staffed by fewer staff unable to attend to even the basic needs of service users is a context of deteriorating health among older people in care.[48]

The centralisation of care provision into a smaller number of larger companies is leading to the growth of larger residential homes which has already been shown to be lowering the quality of care. The most prominent recent example of both of these tendencies is the scandal of abuse of people with learning disabilities at Winterbourne View residential home. The abuse, exposed in 2011, graphically illustrates the decline in both the quality and quantity of residential care for people with learning disabilities in particular, as well as illustrating many of the issues involved in the move to fewer, larger institutions across the sector generally. Sir Stephen Bubb, who led the investigation into the abuse, said: 'It is outrageous that in the 21st century we still treat people with learning disabilities and autism in this appalling way – seclusion, restraint, injections. It is unacceptable.'[49]

Following Winterbourne View, the Care Quality Commission carried out a national survey of learning disability provision in England which showed generally very poor standards of care. Significantly, the audit showed that in terms of the quality of care and length of stay, community-based NHS provision was much better than that provided privately, despite decades of successive governments seeking to build private provider capacity. For profit-driven independent sector care providers larger units allow for economies of scale, underpinning the supervision of more residents by fewer staff and contextualising the decline in standards of care exemplified by Winterbourne View.

Partly in response to the abject failure of independent sector care provision and driven by general commodity market constraints to centralise capital in fewer, larger hands, various UK government-backed schemes have been launched to link social care provision with new forms of extended, privatised healthcare. In other words, the policy solution for the failure of the market in social care has been to encourage their replacement by a smaller number of much larger ones stretching across the traditional health and social care divide. From 2014 in the UK the government trialled ways of doing this, attempting to develop models through 'vanguard' projects, whereby one agency or partnership of agencies can be funded by governments via local authorities to take on the full responsibility of providing all social care. Some 23 vanguard sites are developing new, population-based models for local health services. MCP and PACS vanguards are aiming to bring together budgets and more closely integrate NHS services and social care. For example, the MCP care model is described as a 'new type of integrated provider' which aims to combine the delivery of primary care and community-based healthcare services. Importantly, this will include providing 'some services currently based in hospitals, such as some outpatient clinics or care for frail older people, as well as diagnostics and day surgery'.[50] In other words MCPs are vehicles for shifting some NHS provision into the independent sector for private capital to run at a profit. Public Assistance Committees (PACs) are a form of non-hospital-based private healthcare provision, which are seemingly expanded versions of MCPs.

While some of the vanguards continue to use informal partnerships to take forward their plans, commissioners and providers in many areas are putting in place more formal governance arrangements – in some cases describing the new arrangements as integrated care organisations or accountable care organisations or systems. As they prepare to contract for the new models, many commissioners and providers are considering which entity or partnership should hold a whole population budget and the relationship it should have with other services in complex local systems. For example, in 2017 Manchester's NHS and social care commissioners offered a tender of £6 billion over ten years for a single organisation to provide all 'out of hospital' healthcare provision.[51]

In the UK, the privatisation of healthcare grinds on, driven by a combination of economic requirements, employers' needs to ensure a relatively healthy workforce fit enough to work, an ideological belief in the superiority of a health market to deliver this and a belief that health represents a new area of potential profit. Politically, given the huge popularity – and effectiveness – of the state-run, free at the point of delivery model of healthcare the UK has enjoyed for the past 60 years, fully imposing market relations on healthcare services continues to prove difficult for governments, with numerous local campaigns defending local hospitals and national campaigns coming together in support of the NHS model. Yet governments persist, even when, as we have seen, the market model breaks down and fails to provide a care service adequate for the task. In a sense, UK governments have little choice unless they choose to buck the trend entirely and challenge the dominance of neoliberal polity. As I explain in Chapter 3, the dominant paradigm in healthcare provision, and with regard to health more generally, is that of the commodification of health within the context of competitive market relations of healthcare. Until the dominance of that paradigm is ended those in control of UK healthcare provision must compete in this global market or be outmanoeuvred by other providers.

3

Mergers, Monopolies and the 'Rising Billions'

Health is no more of a priority of the American health system than safe, cheap, efficient, pollution-free transportation is a priority of the American automobile industry.[1]

In 2018 average life expectancy in the US fell for the second year in a row.[2] This is alarming because life expectancy has risen for much of the past century in developed countries, including the US. The decline in US health relative to other countries, however, is not new – it has been unfolding for decades. In 1960, Americans had the highest life expectancy, 2.4 years higher than the average for countries in the Organisation for Economic Co-operation and Development (OECD). But the US started losing ground in the 1980s. US life expectancy fell below the OECD average in 1998, plateaued in 2012, and is now 1.5 years lower than the OECD average (see Figure 3.1).[3] As this chapter shows, this decline correlates almost exactly with the rise to prominence and the seemingly unstoppable increase in wealth of the US private health industry, termed the medical–industrial complex in the 1960s by the Health Policy Advisory Centre, a collection of health activists at the time demanding better healthcare.

Healthcare in the US is in a seemingly intractable state of crisis, failing to provide adequate care for the majority and hugely expensive for those who can afford insurance premiums which have increased wildly over the last decade. The US is a world leader in the concepts of health as a commodity bought on the market and paid for through insurance. Over 45,000 people die each year because they can't afford health insurance.[4] A survey in 2016 found that 52 per cent of Americans can't afford more than $100 per month on health insurance, an amount likely to buy bare-bones coverage only.[5] It is also a political hot potato, as the results of the 2018 mid-term elections in the US showed. There

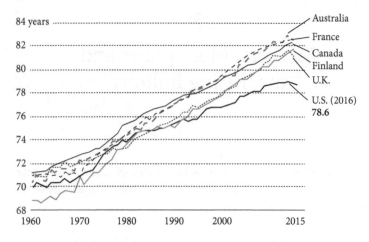

Figure 3.1 US life expectancies decline and fall behind OECD average

was a huge swing of votes away from Trump's Republican Party, which had spent two years attacking the Affordable Care Act, or 'Obamacare', a relatively moderate scheme to support some to be able to buy healthcare insurance. A Reuters/Ipsos poll conducted in the immediate aftermath of the elections showed that healthcare was the top issue on the minds of Democratic and independent voters. As Bill Galston, veteran of six presidential campaigns said, 'In the midterms they were much more the pro-health insurance party than they were the anti-Trump party.'[6]

This is the last in a series of battles to improve US healthcare access that has been opposed by the major health industry corporations. Health sociologist John Geyman adds: 'The corporate, largely privatized market-based U.S. health care system is deteriorating in terms of increasing costs, decreasing access, unacceptable quality of care, inequities, and disparities. Reform efforts to establish universal insurance coverage have failed on six occasions over the last century, largely through opposition of corporate stakeholders in the medical-industrial complex.'[7] In the US, if you can't afford health coverage there are two broad safety nets, Medicare and Medicaid. These are government-run programmes which evolved over the course of the 1960s, in response to failing healthcare systems and mass upheavals in American society, then in the midst of the civil rights movement, the beginnings of anti-Vietnam war revolts and other social unrest. The schemes formed part of President Lyndon Johnson's so-called 'Great Society' projects, a partial acknowledgement in the midst of this social upheaval that governments needed to do something to meet the healthcare needs of its population. The social and political upheavals of the 1960s were key in setting the context for the passing into law of Medicare and Medicaid. During this period the phrase 'medical–industrial complex' came into being, coined by a leading member of one of the many health activists' groups, the Health Policy Advisory Centre, or Health/PAC, to describe the network of US and multinational corporations taking control of healthcare services and health commodities. Health/PAC documented how in the early 1960s powerful New York City teaching hospitals had been granted lucrative affiliation contracts by the municipal governments to provide teaching at the city's run-down public hospitals. Health/PAC argued the teaching hospitals ignored the public health needs of working-class communities local to them, regarding them merely as research guinea pigs. The period was one of intense community activism in New York and elsewhere. For example, the Lincoln Hospital, then known locally as 'the butcher's shop', was occupied by the Black Panthers and Young Lords, two prominent civil and human rights activists groups, resulting in immediate improvements in the service there.[8] Medicare developed as part of this period of protest. It provides health coverage to people aged 65 and older and for those who have a disability, no matter what your income is, through a national programme administered state by state. It most closely equates to what Europeans might call social care.

Similarly, Medicaid provides health coverage if you have a very low income and have no insurance of your own. In terms of residential accommodation for, in particular, older people needing social care, most Americans who enter residential homes do so as private payers, spending their assets until they qualify for coverage from Medicaid. Residential care home places and home care (called In-Home Health Aide) are expensive. According to *Forbes* magazine, in 2016 In-House Health Aide cost an average of $3,800 per month, an annual cost of over $46,000. For a nursing home place the average annual cost for a 'semi-private' room is in excess of $82,000.[9] Costs have nearly doubled since 2013. As a result, it does not take long for many Americans to use up any personal wealth and qualify for Medicaid assistance.[10] The systems interlink. Medicare covers a limited number of days only for nursing home care for rehabilitative services, usually after discharge from hospital. If people need care beyond the Medicare limit, they must pay privately or qualify for

Medicaid coverage. In 2015, Medicare provided health insurance for over 55 million people – 46 million aged 65 and older and nine million younger, disabled people.[11] On average, Medicare covers about half of healthcare charges; the other half must be paid for by individuals themselves. If you can't pay, you aren't covered.

Obamacare was one response to a genuine crisis of ill health – and poverty-related ill health – stalking the US. Low-wage workers are most often not offered health insurance at work or are offered plans that are too expensive or too skimpy.[12] Most of the low-wage jobs that potential Medicaid recipients could obtain do not provide health insurance. In the context described above of ever-increasing care costs, uninsured older people will need to draw increasingly on the Medicaid budget. According to the 2014 Medical Expenditure Panel Survey, only 28 per cent of employees of private firms with low average wages (e.g. retail, food service, agriculture) get health insurance through their jobs.[13] Expanding and deepening poverty in the 'richest country in the world', and the ill health that accompanies it, is the social crisis that underlies the crisis in healthcare. Over 15 per cent – nearly 46 million people – live below the poverty line in the US, representing a vast army of unemployed and low-paid workers unprotected by any kind of healthcare provision.[14]

Even when low-wage businesses offer insurance, workers are often ineligible because they work part time or have not been on the job long enough. When job-based insurance is available, the monthly premiums are frequently too high to be affordable or have such high deductibles that they do not offer meaningful access to care.[15] Obamacare helps low-wage workers move from public to private coverage if their job opportunities expand and incomes rise. Under Obamacare, when earnings rise above the Medicaid income eligibility level workers are deemed able to afford private insurance. Workers are given a subsidy to enable them to buy insurance, in effect passing on this subsidy to the insurance companies and saving the government money in potentially expensive Medicare payouts. US employers have a genuine need to devise a means by which these tens of millions of low-paid workers are kept healthy enough to continue to work. Interruptions in the supply of workers for retail, agriculture, care work and the rest, can cause labour shortages and the potential for resultant wage hikes. Donald Trump's nationalism, trade tariffs and political-ideological attack on migrant workers – a key resource for all of these industries – may, in fact, exacerbate the need for a healthy indigenous workforce.

A second factor for the instability in US healthcare and one of the reasons health is at the centre of political debate are the rising costs of its various elements – drugs, healthcare services, residential care, insurance payments and so on.[16] The US spends more on health than any other country in the world. In 2015, US healthcare spending increased by 5.8 per cent to reach $3.2 trillion, or $9,990 per person.[17] Alongside this, rising poverty meant more people had to rely on Medicaid, while the price of drugs continues to rise. Drug production has been 'financialised'.[18] Leading drugs companies, such as Valeant Pharmaceuticals, have turned away from expensive and relatively unprofitable drug development, instead focusing on mergers and acquisitions. Valeant has developed a three-pronged strategy to do this – acquisition, price gouging and tax avoidance. Typically, Valeant acquires a competitor producing a similar drug to theirs. Once bought, staff cuts, reductions in money spent on research and other savings are made. Now a monopoly holder of a particular drug type, prices are increased. For example, after acquiring the drug Glumetza, used in diabetes, its price increased from just over $500 to $4,400 per month. Finally, in an example of perfectly legal but ethically questionable tax avoidance, Valeant executed an 'inversion' takeover with a Canadian firm, placing the taxable centre of the company in a relatively cheaper tax area. Consequently, as health customers pay more the company pays out less.[19]

The overall share of the US economy devoted to healthcare spending was 17.8 per cent in 2015, up from 17.4 per cent in 2014. The US spends nearly a fifth of its GDP on health and the trend is further upwards. This compares with 9.1 per cent in the UK, 11.2 per cent in Germany, 5.5 per cent in China and 4.7 per cent in India (all figures for 2014).[20] The huge cost of US healthcare is serviced by individual expenditure, with the average 'healthcare consumer' now facing far higher medical costs. Between 2010 and 2015, employees' contributions to health insurance grew almost three times faster than wages. Recent research showed that so-called 'middle-class' Americans are feeling this burden the most – their healthcare spending as a percentage of household income has increased 60 per cent since the 1990s with their healthcare costs now almost half of a typical mortgage payment.[21] Americans are going into debt to service health insurance, spreading health debt to the financial sector.[22]

The rising cost of healthcare is not bad news for everyone, however. Share prices in health-related industries have soared. In 2017 three vast health conglomerates were in the top ten of the US Fortune 500. As a result, US health industries have never been as powerful, or as rich. In 2017, the three health companies were each richer than former market giants General Motors and AT&T. Health market leader McKesson is a pharmaceutical distributor also concerned with the development and distribution of health technologies – a kind of health Walmart. United Health, largely a health insurance provider, has, it is estimated, over 100 million customers globally.

An accelerating context of mergers and acquisitions (M&As) has accompanied and facilitated this enriching process.[23] The tendency for companies to merge into a smaller number of large, industry-specific companies is part of industrial capitalism's DNA. It is currently very much in evidence in health industries globally. Health industry mergers in the US have been accelerating over the last 10 to 15 years. The total reported deal value of M&As in the US health industry in 2016 was $71.7 billion. That was down 59.6 per cent from 2015, the record year for M&As in the sector when the figure, in excess of $100 billion, was equivalent to over a third of the total UK GDP for that year.[24] This process has been described as 'paradigmatic of "Third Wave Capitalism"', with monopoly ownership of health businesses, characterised by interlocking relationships between business and government, blurring the lines between for-profit and not-for-profit entities.[25] Marxists have described M&As as a process of the 'centralisation of capital', the coming together of individual capitalists into fewer, larger conglomerates. In the US the trend towards, and the capitalists' rationale for, actively promoting and pursuing M&As was outlined at the beginning of the twenty-first century, when it was argued that 'facing the drivers of change – deteriorating public health, poor quality and safety, and unaffordable healthcare – the industry is poised to experience convergence among the major suppliers'.[26] 'Poor quality and safety' here refers to the fact that US hospitals increasingly represent a danger to your health. In 2013 medical errors in hospitals were the leading cause of preventable death in the country, accounting for nearly a quarter of all preventable deaths that year, beating smoking and obesity-related illness into second and third place as the 'butcher shop' approach to public hospitals returns.[27] In 2005 it was estimated that there were over 98,000 preventable deaths each year in US hospitals, costing the system over \$38 billion annually.[28]

The monopolising centralisation of health capital is not restricted, of course, to the US alone – it is a global phenomenon. Global expansion is, in fact, another driver of US health industry growth and finance is currently being sucked into the health industry as never before by the promise of the growing potential of a global market in ill health, euphemistically called the 'rising billions' driven by technological change.[29] This is the idea that over the immediate future between three and five billion new consumers worldwide will be connected to the internet for the first time, greatly expanding the medical–industrial complex's potential catalogue of 'health customers'. eHealth systems also represent a technology-driven growth area for the medical–industrial complex in the US as elsewhere. eHealth covers a broad field including systems of communication between health practitioners, remote health monitoring and virtual consultations between doctors, other professionals and patients. At a more mundane level, by 2018 hospitals were cutting costs by using household drills instead of specialised surgical ones, and mosquito netting instead of surgical mesh for internal organ repair.[30]

In the 1870s Marx analysed the drive towards technological advance inherent in capitalism. He argued that labour-saving machinery produced in this way could potentially eliminate arduous work for future societies, potentially freeing humankind for more creative activity.[31] However, as Marx was at great pains to point out, as long as a tiny minority of the population continued to own the means of production – factories, machinery, even the production of ideas through schools and universities – technological advance would not be used in this way. Instead, technological advance has typically been used to make some workers redundant while making those left work harder, increasing their rate of exploitation. The length of our working day, how quickly we are made to work and the overall productivity of our labour are ways in which technological change facilitates this increased exploitation and increased profit for the employer. In the global health industry, manipulation of all three of these has been evident, in differing combinations in different geopolitical circumstances for decades now. In the US, UK and elsewhere healthcare staff are in short supply. Research in the US, for example, shows that another 2.3 million workers are needed over the next five years in order to keep up with demand. Wages in the US are low, with care staff earning less than $12 per hour and nursing assistants $13, nowhere near enough to afford the soaring costs of health insurance.[32] Technological advance, even in healthcare with such obvious reliance on labour-intensive methodologies, in time-honoured tradition is being used not to improve the quality of care or make work easier but to squeeze more out of fewer workers.

Marx and before him Adam Smith were very precise about what was meant by 'exploitation'. Importantly, exploitation doesn't mean you are being treated extraordinarily unfairly. Exploitation is central to the processes by which profit is ordinarily generated:

> As soon as stock has accumulated in the hands of particular persons, some of them will naturally employ it in setting to work industrious people, whom they will supply with materials and subsistence, in order to make a profit by the sale of their work, or by what their labour adds to the value of the materials ... The value which the workmen add to the materials, therefore, resolves itself in this case into two parts, of which one pays their wages, the other the profits of their employer upon the whole stock of materials and wages which he advanced.[33]

For Smith, workers 'add value' through this process of exploitation and this value is realised as profit. Deepening exploitation has implications for healthcare users but also for healthcare workers and their health. As I discuss in Chapter 4, employment is a central aspect of what has become known as the social determinants of health approach. How, how hard and in what conditions we work have profound effects on an individual's health, and this has been the case since the inception of industrial capitalism in the late eighteenth century. As Smith shows, this process of exploitation is the essential element of capitalist production, and as he and (later and in more detail) Marx showed, increasing the rates of exploitation is endemic. Capitalist employment is no more than systematised exploitation – when WHO says that work potentially has detrimental effects on our health, in effect they are saying that the process of exploitation central to capitalist production makes us ill. We might say that this process of exploitation produces a health deficit that, although working people have historically found ways of ameliorating it, we can never fully address so long as we remain wage labourers. The dominant health paradigm described here – of health as a commodity for sale on a healthcare market – locks this health deficit in.

These considerations are of little concern to the brokers on Wall Street and elsewhere dealing in health stocks and shares. The 'health bubble' thus produced is making at least some very nervous:

> What is larger than the UK's entire economy, soaring in price, wildly profitable, the leading cause of personal bankruptcy, bankrupting the United States and a massive economic bubble that nobody has heard of yet? Healthcare in America ... a modern-day gold rush is on as young Americans clamour for healthcare careers in the same way that young adults were jockeying for technology careers at the peak of the Dot-com bubble in 1999.[34]

The threat of a health bubble collapse makes previous industry collapses – like those in the US auto and building industries – seem like child's play in comparison. The US auto industry contributes around 3.5 per cent of US GDP and employs 1.7 million people. This industry was deemed 'too big to fail' so the US government bailed it out, investing around $80 billion from 2009 to 2014 to keep it from collapsing. Healthcare is five times larger than the auto industry in terms of its percentage contribution to GDP and is ten times larger in terms of the number of people it employs. It's estimated that any comparative bailout of the health industry would cost the government upwards of $400 billion.[35]

As public–private lines blur, the health industry has a parasitic relationship with the US state, being dependent on it to open up new international markets. US military interventions around the globe have made areas 'safe' for health industry expansion. Countries including Iraq and Afghanistan, others in the Middle East and parts of Africa are considered to be regions ripe for US health industry investment.

Writing in 1917, the Marxist Russian Revolutionary Nikolai Bukharin wrote:

> In the epoch of finance capitalism ... the centre of gravity is shifted to the competition of gigantic, consolidated and organised economic bodies possessed of a colossal fighting capacity in the world tournament of 'nations'. Here competition holds its orgies on the greatest possible scale, and together with this there goes on a change

and a shift to a higher phase in the process of capital centralisation. The absorption of small capital units by large ones, the absorption of weak trusts, the absorption even of large trusts by larger ones is relegated to the rear and looks like child's play compared with the absorption of whole countries that are being forcibly torn away from their economic centres and included in the economic system of the victorious 'nation'.[36]

Writing as world war raged around him, Bukharin was able to conceptualise where monopoly capitalism leads. In the twenty-first century, the interests of the US state are in many ways already partially fused with those of the US health industry and the finance capital driving its expansion, and together these contextualise an increasingly impoverished home country and the increasing subjugation of foreign lands. A collapse of the US health industry would be disastrous for US capital generally, threatening jobs and amassed fortunes alike, and providing the potential for fear and frustration to express itself in myriad ways. Meanwhile the profitability of the US medical sector is teetering on the razor edge of a globalised eHealth promise. In this neoliberal scramble for profitability, as we have seen, the health of populations comes a poor second. In a society where health is bought and sold, the possession of a greater quantity of resources ensures better health. This is clearly expressed in disparities in life expectancies between rich and poor, and in ever-widening more general health inequality.

This biomedically defined health paradigm governed by the medical–industrial complex, where health is a commodity to be bought and sold on an increasingly cut-throat neoliberal health market, sits in stark contrast to concepts emanating from WHO, researchers and academics with regard to how health is achieved. An approach to health based on the many and varied social determinants of health potentially opens up debate, presenting a challenge to the dominant, commodity-focused paradigm. It is to an exploration of the strengths and weaknesses of this approach that we now turn.

4

The Social Determinants of Health

The social determinants of health are a combination of social, economic and political factors that shape the health of individuals, communities and populations. These influences determine to a great extent people's state of health or illness. The social determinants of health are overwhelmingly shaped by policy and political ideologies. The WHO says, 'This unequal distribution of health-damaging experiences is not in any sense a "natural" phenomenon but is the result of a toxic combination of poor social policies, unfair economic arrangements and bad politics.'[1]

With regard to acting upon these determinants, two areas of action in particular were recommended by the WHO Commission on the Social Determinants of Health in their 2008 report, *Closing the Gap in a Generation*. The first area that needs addressing is daily living conditions, including healthy physical environments, fair employment and decent work, social protection across the lifespan and access to healthcare. The second major area concerns the distribution of power, money and resources, including equity in health programmes, public financing of action on the social determinants and economic inequalities.[2]

Following *Closing the Gap*, the 2011 World Conference on Social Determinants of Health brought together delegations from 125 member states and resulted in the Rio Political Declaration on Social Determinants of Health. This declaration involved an affirmation that health inequities are unacceptable, and noted that these inequities arise from the societal conditions in which people are born, grow, live, work and age, including early childhood development, education, economic status, employment and decent work, housing environment and effective prevention and treatment of health problems.[3]

Closing the Gap was the most detailed account of the nature and implications of the social determinants of health approach to that point. It suggests various strategies for improving global health through the use of the social determinant methodologies and calls on political powers globally to act to promote the health of their populations. It has gone some way to establishing a basic premise that health is determined socially, by the ways the societies in which we live are structured. As the document argued:

> Traditionally, society has looked to the health sector to deal with its concerns about health and disease. Certainly, maldistribution of healthcare – not delivering care to those who most need it – is one of the social determinants of health. But the high burden of illness responsible for appalling premature loss of life arises in large part because of the conditions in which people are born, grow, live, work, and age.[4]

The 'traditional' view outlined above continues to dominate, concentrating resources on funding for hospitals and medical research on medical techniques and technologies. This approach continues to shape and is itself shaped by ideologies with regard to the medical profession's dominant role in overseeing global health. In its place the commission responsible for *Close the Gap* – which included Michael Marmot, Amartya Sen and other academics and public health experts – seeks to establish a 'holistic' view, pointing to the ways in which we experience health and how ill health is shaped by the conditions in which we live.[5]

Debates about our health have been dominated by biomedical models that have in effect largely confined the debate to one centred on an individual's relationship with natural disease, ameliorated by the expertise of the medical profession. The approach has been dominated by the medical profession and medical industry, and models of healthcare that prioritise those institutionalised ways of managing our health. For the multifaceted approach to health outlined by WHO and others over the early part of this century, the solutions to poor and unequal health outcome expectations lies not simply in global societies ensuring good health service provision, which is one among many health determinants, but in addressing the 'conditions in which people are born, grow, live, work, and age'.[6] In turn this requires the active involvement of 'whole of government, civil society and local communities, business, global fora, and international agencies. Policies and programmes must embrace all the key sectors of society not just the health sector'.[7]

The extent to which societies determine aspects of our health is analysed with great insight by Canguilhem, who shows how little there is about our human make-up that can be considered purely 'natural'. Even something as seemingly purely physical as blood pressure is, he argues, in fact deeply determined by the societies and cultural surroundings in which we live.[8] His body of work illustrates that our physical make-up is deeply influenced by the social, cultural and political contexts we find ourselves in.[9] It argues that our health evolves as a process through our relationships with the types of societies in which we live.

The condition of our global environment, of course, contextualises all analysis of how healthy specific elements of societies – some of which I consider below – may or may not be. There is a great deal of research, not directly the subject of this book, which shows that our environment is becoming more of a threat to general health. A few examples are necessary, however, to provide some global context. A WHO report in 2018[10] shows that poisonous air is having a devastating impact on billions of children around the world, potentially undermining their intellectual growth and leading to hundreds of thousands of deaths. The study found that more than 90 per cent of the world's young people – 1.8 billion children – are breathing toxic air, storing up a public health time bomb for the next generation. WHO said medical experts in almost every field of children's health are uncovering new evidence of the scale of the crisis in both rich and poor countries – from low birth weight to poor neurodevelopment, asthma to heart disease. Dr Tedros Adhanom, WHO's director general, said: 'Polluted air is poisoning millions of children and ruining their lives. This is inexcusable – every child should be able to breathe clean air so they can grow and fulfil their potential.'[11]

Since the end of World War II more than 85,000 new industrial chemicals have been produced and released into the environment with minimal testing or government oversight. Toxic waste is an ever-present by-product of industrial production, with over 200 million people worldwide directly exposed to toxic waste and millions more indirectly exposed.[12] For example, every part of the oil extraction industry – the activity that fuels every other industry – is hazardous to health due to spills, leaks, collision-related fires and burning excess methane and other gases at oil wells, rigs and refineries. All of these risks have the potential to release carbon emissions into the air, contributing to global pollution and climate change. Even emissions from so-called 'cleaner fuels' like natural gas contribute to illness such as asthma, chronic bronchitis, cancers and blood disorders. It is estimated that almost 500,000 premature deaths in Europe alone are caused by air pollution, with air pollution the main cause of death in 41 European countries.[13] Research in the UK found that air pollution was as bad for pregnant women as smoking, raising the risk of miscarriage.[14] An inquest in south London in 2014 found that the death of one young girl from 'severe asthma' was due to the 'unlawfully high levels of pollution' in that part of the capital, the first but unlikely to be the last such court ruling.[15] According to a *Lancet* commission on pollution and health nine million premature deaths, 16 per cent of the world's total, are caused by diseases caused by pollution.[16]

To many of you the idea that our health is influenced by the environment and at a micro level by where we live and by the conditions we live in will not come as a shock. Most of us will be aware that living in damp housing makes you more likely to suffer from respiratory problems, allergies or asthma. We might also be aware that damp and mould impacts on the immune system. Housing has a huge impact on our mental health and well-being too. For example, children living in crowded homes are much more likely to be stressed, anxious, depressed, have poorer physical health and do less well at school.[17] The issue of adequate housing is of course not a new issue. In fact, in the UK governments only paid sufficient attention to providing adequate housing during a relatively short period after World War II. For decades after World War II the UK built on average more than 300,000 new homes a year. In the twenty-first century governments have managed about half that. A decade ago, the Barker Review of Housing Supply noted that about 250,000 homes needed to be built every year to prevent spiralling house prices and a shortage of affordable homes. That target has been consistently missed – the closest the UK got was in 2006–7 when 219,000 homes were built. In 2012–13 the UK hit a post-war low of 135,500 homes, much of which was due to the financial crisis.[18]

The extreme consequence of this is that homelessness is increasing. Since 2010 homelessness in the UK has rocketed, with a national total up 169 per cent since that year, and some 59,000 people officially recognised as homeless.[19] The average life expectancy of a homeless person in the UK in 2018 was 47.[20] According to research from UCL, in the UK homeless people have a higher risk of physical and mental health problems, they are more likely to die from cancer or commit suicide and they have higher rates of alcohol and substance misuse, smoking and tuberculosis.[21] In 2019 homelessness in Oxford became a national scandal when five homeless people died in quick succession on Oxford's streets.[22]

Rates of respiratory disease, tuberculosis, meningitis and gastric conditions are higher in overcrowded households.[23] Overcrowding can impede children's education, family relationships, and physical, mental and emotional well-being.[24] For all age groups, living in a cold, damp home leads to a higher risk of cardiovascular and respiratory diseases, and mental health problems.[25]

In the UK, individuals and couples 'stalled' in the parental home is an increasingly important issue given the lack of affordable housing to buy or rent. In 2017, the Royal Institution of Chartered Surveyors predicted that rents were likely to increase by 25 per cent to 2022, with housing costs up by around 20 per cent, way ahead of any predicted wage inflation for the period.[26] A report published in 2018 shows that the chances of a young adult on a middle income owning a home in the UK have more than halved in the past two decades. The Institute for Fiscal Studies shows how an explosion in house prices above income growth has robbed the younger generation of the ability to buy their own home. For 25–34 year olds earning between £22,200 and £30,600 per year, home ownership fell to just 27 per cent in 2016 from 65 per cent two decades ago. Middle-income young adults born in the late 1980s are now no more likely than those lower down the pay scale to own their own home. Just one in four middle-income young adults own their own home – down from two in three 20 years ago.[27] Of course, if you are able to buy your own home the potentially health-depleting stress doesn't end. The costs of the upkeep of houses along with the pressures of a mortgage and other debt continue to exert a negative health influence. In 2017, analysis of nearly 40,000 research papers into debt and risk to mental health conclusively showed a strong correlation.[28] Meanwhile, living space and the average size of new builds has fallen dramatically. Research in the UK in 2018 showed that the average size of a living room had fallen from 24.9 square metres in the 1970s to 17.1 square metres in 2018, a contraction of 32 per cent.[29] Research found that at an average of 76 square metres in total, the UK's newly built homes were the smallest by floor space in Europe, some way behind the next worst in Italy at 81.5 square metres.[30]

For unemployed people, those in 'in-work poverty', low wages and zero hour contracts getting support for housing costs has been made more difficult by decades of cutbacks. As part of austerity-driven benefits agendas in the UK, housing benefit payments for unemployed people and those on low incomes have been capped, while security of tenure has been reduced giving landlords a freer hand to raise rents, increasing the anxiety of getting and holding on to rented accommodation.[31] Without decisive action in the UK, crowded homes – and the many and varied physical and mental health conditions they bring with them – are set to stay with us for the foreseeable future.

Chronic shortages of adequate housing is a global problem. In the rapidly urbanising cities of LMICs, accommodation is a pressing issue with hundreds of millions of people living in substandard housing, without electricity, running water or basic sanitation. It is estimated that the global affordable housing gap is currently 330 million urban households, and it is forecast to grow by more than 30 per cent to 440 million households, or 1.6 billion people, by 2025.[32] The continued global growth of urban areas and urban populations creates huge demand for land, leading to escalating housing costs, competition and rampant price inflation globally as landlords and housing providers seek to profit from their properties.[33] In China, for example, the World Bank has estimated that the urban population has risen from 19.6 per cent of the population in 1980 to a massive 56 per cent in 2015, creating huge demand and need for affordable housing. According to research, global house prices have risen by over 600 per cent since the beginning of the twenty-first century.[34] The decline in publicly funded properties, a consequence of the running down of the state sector generally identified with neoliberalism, leaves a housing market largely unmanaged or ameliorated by state housing provision or even government policy. A context of fewer, smaller households, more expensive to rent or buy, falls far short of WHO's desire for good quality housing supportive of health.

Diet is another and seemingly obvious social determinant of health long recognised as key. For example, writing in the 1840s Frederick Engels noted:

> Nearly all workers have stomachs more or less weak and are yet forced to adhere to the diet which is the root of the evil … new disease arises during childhood from impaired digestion. Scrofula [a form of tuber-

culosis] is almost universal among the working-class, and scrofulous parents have scrofulous children ... A second consequence of this insufficient bodily nourishment, during the years of growth and development, is rachitis [rickets] which is extremely common among the working-class. The hardening of the bones is delayed, the development of the skeleton in general restricted and deformities of the legs and spinal column are frequent.[35]

From the very birth of industrial capitalism then, doctors, scientists and social commentators of all kinds recognised diet's key determining influence on health. Yet how many times have you visited a doctor with an illness and been asked about your diet? Generally speaking this kind of conversation is not part of the medical discourse in which doctors ordinarily engage. Constrained by a biomedical approach, the majority of doctors will tend to avoid discussion of such socially determined influences on health as diet, housing and the like. Yet susceptibility to diseases of all kinds are contextualised by diet and how they support or disable immune systems. Tuberculosis (TB) is a pathogenic bacteria which has been identified in prehistoric remains. It remains a global threat today, impacting especially upon the poor and those made vulnerable by poor living conditions and diet.[36] TB rates in the UK fell after – and during – World War II, as for many diet, healthcare and housing improved. In 2015, Public Health England named TB as one its health priorities in greatest need of improvement, along with smoking, obesity, alcohol and dementia, as the incidence of TB rises.[37]

Readers will be aware of at least some of the deficiency or excess dietary-related problems, such as obesity and eating disorders, and chronic diseases such as cardiovascular disease, hypertension, cancer and diabetes mellitus that are common modern-day illnesses linked to twenty-first century diets. You might also be aware that these disorders are unequally distributed in the population as a whole, affecting working-class, and especially poorer working-class people disproportionately.[38] In the US unhealthy diets directly contribute to approximately 678,000 deaths every year,[39] though the indirect contribution of poor diet to early and avoidable death is not calculable. The so-called 'junk food epidemic' hangs over modern life. In 2000, US citizens spent $110 billion on junk food, more than on higher education or on the cinema, books, magazines, newspapers, videos and recorded music combined.[40]

Research in Karnataka, India, found that increased junk food consumption there had led to increases in obesity, food poisoning, dehydration and arthritis among other ailments and diseases.[41] The UK has one of the highest prevalences of obesity in Europe at 25 per cent, and the number of people living with type 2 diabetes has more than doubled since 1996. Both cost the NHS £16 billion a year, and the UK economy at large £47 billion a year in treatment costs and lost working hours.[42] Yet government responses have focused on developing treatments and cures, rather than on ways of preventing diet-related illness in the first place, a curative rather than preventative approach that privileges the medical–industrial complex and the dominant 'health as a commodity' paradigm explained earlier.

Food adulteration, where inferior substances are added or valuable ingredients of food are removed, remains an important health concern. The situation has changed slightly since the nineteenth century and early UK capitalism when 'the refuse of soap-boiling establishments … [was] mixed with other things and sold as sugar … Cocoa is often adulterated with fine brown earth, treated with fat to render it more easily mistakable for real cocoa'.[43] But it has not changed as much as we might think. Today, so-called 'economically motivated adulteration', or 'food fraud', has consistently shown how inadequate regulatory systems for food standards are worldwide, how ruthless the food industry can be and how potentially dangerous these practices are.[44]

Increasingly globalised food supply chains and the economic motivation to provide cheaper food products have contributed to food fraud. According to NSF International's Global Food Safety Division Managing Director David Edwards:

What we're seeing today is an increasingly complex and fragmented food supply chain. Due to both its global nature and the fact that most food today no longer follows a straight line from source to fork, it is more like a supply 'network,' and tracing an ingredient back to its source has become challenging due to this increasing network of handlers, suppliers and middlemen globally.[45]

In addition to the globalisation of the supply network making detection harder and adulteration easier, other trends influencing the rise in food fraud include cost cutting, as the food industry is under constant pressure to keep prices down. That leads to the temptation to substitute.

In the UK the food and drink industry is worth in excess of £200 billion per year and, as such, is 'vulnerable to a wide range of criminal activity'.[46] For example, the Food Crime Unit's annual report of 2016 shows cases of pet food being diverted into the human food chain, species substitution – lamb for beef, turkey or pork – and animal waste products being channelled into human consumption pathways.[47] Older readers will remember the salmonella scare of 1988, when it was found that the poor animal welfare practices of factory farm chickens was causing the deadly virus to be found in eggs. It took another 30 years, until October 2017, for the UK's Food Standards Agency to declare all Lion Mark eggs to be officially salmonella free.[48] Again, as with housing, this is clearly not just a UK problem. In 2011 in China, melamine adulteration of infant formula resulted in over 300,000 serious illnesses, with unpredictable long-term costs to the children's health.[49] In 2017, contaminated eggs from a Dutch farm spread out over Europe, with the UK, Denmark, Belgium and Germany among others forced to withdraw foodstuffs from sale.[50]

The world's total food and drinks supply is controlled by ten mega-conglomerates – Nestlé, PepsiCo, Coca-Cola, Unilever, Danone, General Mills, Kellogg's, Mars, Associated British Foods and Mondelēz – each with annual profits in the tens of billions. They wield unimaginable economic and political power worldwide and present a serious challenge for governments to manage – should governments feel inclined to do so through food standards policies and related legislation. For example, food processor Nestlé's 2007 profits were $9.7 billion, greater than the combined GDP of the 65 poorest countries in the world. As Empson argues, 'Corporations like these dominate agriculture to such an extent that they can alter government policy, prices and drive smaller companies out of business'.[51]

We might want to ask how concerned and consistent governments are in their attempts to control this global behemoth. A report in 2016 cast doubt on successive UK governments' determination in this regard. They show that despite several decades-worth of research showing conclusively that artificially reducing saturated fats in foods is not the inevitable route to good health it is claimed to be and that saturated fat too has a part to play in a balanced diet.[52] The Public Health Collaboration report points to the deteriorating health outcomes of the UK population over this period and asks, 'if the UK had been advised to go for foods in their natural form instead of unnaturally man-made low-fat foods for the past 30 years' then there would not be such an epidemic of diet-related diseases.[53]

Those in positions of power and influence while in government have a documented history of developing close links with the very organisations governments would need to manage to ensure high standards of food, potentially producing conflicts of interest. In the UK, in 2016 Jim Paice, former secretary of state for agriculture and food, was working as director of farming for Camgrain and chairman of dairy giant First Milk Ltd. Former Health Secretary Andrew Lansley advised the giant Swiss drugs firm Roche, private equity giant Blackstone on healthcare investments and management consultants Bain and Co. on 'healthcare innovation'. Roche was one of the main beneficiaries of the Cancer Drugs Fund Lansley set up in 2010.[54] The list of such links is extensive. No fraud is implied here, but it does raise questions regarding government ministers' determination to protect public health by controlling the activities of giant food and health industry firms if they are likely to take up posts in these same industries once they leave office.

Of course, this is not just a UK problem. In the US, Republican Congressman Tom Price was initially appointed as secretary of the huge Health and Human Services department by the incoming Trump administration in 2016. The six-term Georgia Republican was positioned to oversee vast social programmes and have led the Food and Drug Administration (FDA), the Centers for Disease Control and Prevention, the National Institutes of Health and other agencies. The Department of Health and Human Services, with a budget of $1 trillion, is the world's largest source of funding for medical research. Price would have controlled FDA policies regulating drugs, medical devices and diagnostic tests. In the months after his appointment CNN, the *New York Times* and the *Wall Street Journal* all carried stories showing that Price traded more than $300,000 worth of stocks in companies that stood to benefit from legislation he supported or drafted, revelations which subsequently made his position untenable.[55] As I discuss in more detail below, the blurring between the public and private spheres endemic to this phase of capitalism consistently lead to the possibility of abuse of power on a personal level, and the use of state power to benefit private health capital as the expense of the rest of us.

It is not simply the quality and quantity of food that comprises the social determinant that is diet, it is how the supply of that food and drink is organised and managed: what we might call the ownership of the means of food production is problematic at a fundamental level. The extremely small number of individuals and organisations who own the means of producing the food we consume are complicit in the poor health outcomes resultant from our daily diet. To impact on the diets and improve the health outcomes of populations, be they local or global, we need to impact on those who own and run the global food industry. This is an issue discussed in the final report of the Fabian Commission on Food and Poverty, published in 2015. In it they conclude that governments must take 'responsibility for food and household food insecurity back from charities, businesses and individuals. To do this, the UK government should take a lead coordinating role to end household food insecurity.'[56]

Employment – what we do, for how long and in what conditions in order to earn a living – is the final health determinant I will discuss. The workplace has always been the central concern with regard to individual and public health and it remains so in the twenty-first century, feeding into other determinants such as diet and accommodation. The precise nature of the health risks faced by workers may have changed over the centuries – though probably not as much as you might think – but the prevalence and intensity of those risks remain as deadly in their consequences as they ever have been. For example, developing the concept of 'employment strain', Canadian Wayne Lewchuk and others describe the health consequences of a process of casualisation of work:

> Workers in precarious employment relationships report poorer overall health than working Canadians and higher levels of stress ... They face high levels of uncertainty regarding access to work, the terms and conditions of work and future earnings. They engage in additional effort searching for work and balancing the demands of multiple employers. They have low earnings, few benefits and reside in low income households.[57]

This study is a revealing analysis of one aspect of employment over the recent past: the further casualisation and increasing job insecurity of employment which has worked its way into areas of employment previously regarded aas relatively secure, like teaching and local authority employment. It also illustrates how employment feeds into other determinants like diet and accommodation discussed above.

In many parts of the world since the 1980s, call centres have come to dominate how enterprises, public services and organisations interact with customers, clients and the public. Their growth has often coincided with developments in technology and was spurred by the economic and financial crisis of 2008. Since then, the call centre industry has emerged as a distinctive organisational form, transforming the location and nature of customer services internationally. More recently, it has become increasingly prevalent in developing countries.[58] Research into call centre employment in the UK throws light on the health consequences of such work.[59] The report shows that along with the risk of repetitive strain injury common to all twenty-first century office-based work, broader potential problems arise resulting from the combination of keyboard, desk, mouse, screen, headset and voice used together, often under pressure. Research by the Health and Safety Executive (HSE) found significantly higher stress levels in frontline call handlers than in benchmark groups in other occupations. The lack of control staff have over the fast pace and flow of work contributes a great deal to work-related stress and dissatisfaction. HSE guidance also points to 'inappropriate monitoring', or overzealous supervision from team leaders, as a source of stress.[60] The British Unite trade union's guide to health and safety in call centres says that call centre staff turnover can vary anywhere between 20 per cent and 80 per cent a year, and that a large part of this 'burn out' results from stress.[61] The study by the Institute of Occupational Safety and Health found that one in four call centre agents suffer voice problems, including voice loss, sore throats and breathlessness, because managers are failing to protect their health. Up to 60 per cent of workers reported having difficulty making themselves heard against background noise and 41 per cent said they had failed to be heard by the customer on the other end of the line. Researchers found that new starters, especially female workers, were at particularly high risk of ill health.[62]

These insecure and stressful workplace conditions set a context, in the UK and globally, for the rising levels of mental illnesses which are increasingly being recognised as impacting on people's daily work lives. In the UK it is estimated that up to 17 per cent of workers continue at work with some form of mental illness. Nearly half – 43.4 per cent – of UK adults feel they have had some kind of diagnosable mental illness in their lifetimes.[63] Research suggests that in China the enormous shift in populations from rural to urban employment, internal migration and the insecurity and social exclusion it often causes is at the root of the marked increase in mental illness there.

At a global level, the International Labour Organization estimates that around 2.3 million people die each year as a result of work-related accidents, while an additional 270 million people suffer work injuries with a long-term impact on their lives, and 160 million suffer from short- and long-term illness related to their work.[64] It is estimated there are about 250 million child labourers worldwide, that is one in six of all children aged 5 to 17 on the face of the globe, working long hours usually in hazardous conditions.[65] Of these, 179 million – one in every eight – are trapped in the worst forms of labour, endangering their long-term physical, mental and moral well-being. At a global level, the majority of these (70 per cent) are in agriculture, an industry with little or no opportunities for advancement or change.[66] Here are two accounts of agricultural-based child labour:

Much of this labour is of a kind highly injurious to children, requiring a continued stooping posture with a considerable amount of physical effort. Pulling turnips is perhaps the most pernicious employment to which a child can be set; it strains the spine and often lays the foundation of chronic disease ... The turnip leaves in the early morning are often full of ice, which greatly aggravates the sufferings of those employed in the work; the backs of the hands becomes swollen and cracked by the wind and cold and wet, the palms blister, and the fingers bleed from frequent laceration.[67]

The two main activities that may be classified as hazardous in sugar cane cultivation are the application of agro-chemicals for crop protection and manual harvesting, which involves the use of sharp tools. Crop protection exposes children to harmful agro-chemicals, especially pesticides, which can cause respiratory diseases and irritation of the skin or eyes and have long-term consequences such as cancer and neurological damage. Manual harvesting involves many health and safety risks, including injury (due to use of dangerous tools, and insect and snake bites), musculoskeletal disorders (repetitive movements and transportation of heavy loads) and exposure to sunlight, high temperatures and hazardous chemicals.[68]

The first of these comes from a UK Children's Commission report from 1867, the other from an International Labour Organization report of 2017. After 150 years the health risks remain largely the same, only the geography and climate has changed in this case. Employment remains central to distributions of poor health outcomes and to an understanding of health inequalities. Where and how we work has the potential to undermine our health, but also these nodes of social collaboration have the potential to fundamentally address health issues, as I show in Chapter 8.

Inequalities in experiences of housing, diet, education, employment and more are together constituent of health and health inequalities. As such it is useful to understand health inequalities as a conglomerate of other, socially determined, inequalities. The unequal distributions of health illustrate this broad range of other social and political inequalities. Consequently, if we are to impact on our health, we need to make an impact on these other inequalities. For example, finding ways of securing better housing, better diets and better conditions of employment, means we are implicitly finding ways of addressing broader health concerns. Looked at this way, health ceases to be an individualised concern to be negotiated with medical professionals and becomes a collective concern to do with how we work together to improve the material conditions of our lives.

This chapter has detailed an approach to health focused on its social determinants espoused by WHO and others. This, I argue, is a very useful direction to go in, shifting the emphasis onto concerns with addressing the lived social and political contexts of health, way beyond an understanding of health constrained by medical models focused on individuals' bodies in their relationship with disease. In the approach pioneered by WHO, ill health arises as a consequence of poor social and political environments. The cure is not a course of tablets or eating an apple a day, The cure lies in finding ways of improving the material conditions in which we live and work.

5

The 'Inequality Thesis'

This chapter examines the 'inequality thesis', a set of ideas concerned with showing that inequality in health exists, is related to income inequality and has a bad effect on communities and societies generally. The thesis, which evolved over the course of the twenty-first century, has been pioneered by a wide range of academics, including Michael Marmot, Kate Pickett, Richard Wilkinson and Danny Dorling. It has been a fantastically useful one in drawing attention to the growing gap between the health expectations and outcomes of different members of society. Their work has turned the issue of health inequalities into a central concern at the policy and public awareness level, and it should be celebrated in this regard. This chapter seeks to build on this work by examining important elements of the thesis. The body of evidence they, and others, have built over the course of the last decade and more is immense, and this chapter explores what we might add to their analysis by way of critique.

In their pioneering and best-selling book, *The Spirit Level*, Wilkinson and Pickett state that 'Most of us now wish we could eat less rather than more. And for the first time in history the poor are – on average – fatter than the rich. Economic growth, so long the great engine of progress, has, in rich countries, largely finished its work.'[1] I shall return to a detailed analysis of this later in this chapter, but first want to contextualise it by looking at the body of thought the statement is influenced by. Richard Wilkinson in particular has been at the centre of arguments about health inequality throughout the twenty-first century. Representing the general thrust of an academic trend, Wilkinson argues that above a certain level of a country's gross national product per capita the major determinant of health is income inequality. His research shows that in developed countries the greater a nation's income inequality, the poorer the average national health status across the entire population. For Wilkinson, it is inequality rather than wealth that is important for health, not an individual's income but how unequal is the society she or he is living in.

The thrust of *The Spirit Level* is that health inequality is bad for entire societies.

For Wilkinson and others, a focus on absolute levels of income-related determinants of health does not explain why some 'rich' countries show lower levels of average health than do some poorer, but more egalitarian countries. They argue that within countries there are differences in health status across the socio-economic status (SES) gradient. That is, it is not simply poorer people for whom higher rates of ill health are a problem. Even SES groups quite high in income and status show poorer health than those immediately above them, a point made by another great advocate of this approach, Michael Marmot.[2] Wilkinson and other inequality theorists have turned more recently to the indirect influence of psycho-social factors on health rather than simply the direct and immediate effects of material life circumstances. If indeed health is related to social status, then psycho-social factors, not only the material conditions of life, are important. This approach is at odds with the social determinants of health approach discussed earlier. The inequality thesis, though referencing social determinants, uses them in a way that produces a less clearly effective analysis of health outcomes and their causes. How has inequality theory come to this point?

Let us look first at the idea that status is the key determinant of health, most vividly expressed in the early work of Michael Marmot in his Civil Servant Studies, which took place over two phases: in the 1960s and in a follow-up study 20 years later. Whitehall I compared the mortality rates of people in the highly hierarchical environment of the British Civil Service. It showed that among British civil servants, mortality was higher among those in the lower grade when compared to the higher grade. The higher up the employment hierarchy, the longer the life expectancy compared to people in lower grades. Whitehall I found higher mortality rates across a range of causes for men of lower grades. Coronary heart disease was found to be particularly prevalent.[3]

The study found that lower grades were also more likely to be obese, to smoke and to have reduced leisure time, lower levels of physical activity, higher prevalence of underlying illness, higher blood pressure and shorter height. From this Marmot concluded that the lower status of the lower grades was the root cause of health and mortality differences. Twenty years later, the Whitehall II study documented a similar gradient in morbidity in women as well as men.[4] Whitehall II revealed this social gradient across an increased range of diseases including some cancers, chronic lung disease, gastrointestinal disease, depression, suicide and others.[5] It found that the way work is organised, the work climate, social influences outside work, influences from early life and health behaviours all contribute to in-work health inequalities. Subjects of Whitehall II in the lowest employment grades were more likely to have many of the established risk factors of coronary heart disease: a propensity to smoke, lower height-to-weight ratio, less leisure time and higher blood pressure.[6]

The studies are extremely important in indicating the differing health problems and outcomes associated with different types and grades of employment. Its focus on the stressful and often actively unhealthy nature of employment is also a major strength. However, the use of the sociological concept of 'status' used by inequality theorists is problematic.

Status-related sociological theory is rooted in the work of German sociologist Max Weber (1864–1920), who formulated a three-component theory of social stratification that defines a status group as a group of people who, within a society, can be differentiated on the basis of non-economic qualities such as honour, prestige, ethnicity, race and religion. Weber said that status stands in stark contrast with social class, based on economically determined relationships.[7] According to Weber, status groups feature in a wide variety of social stratifications including categorisation by race, ethnicity, caste, professional groups, neighbourhood groups, nationalities and so on. These contrast with relationships rooted in economic relations, or class. As sociologist Anthony Giddens points out, whereas class is objectively given, status 'depends on people's subjective evaluation of social differences. Classes derive from the economic factors associated with property and earnings; status is governed by the varying styles of life groups follow.'[8] The use of status as a central defining feature of health inequality is, then, a subjective approach to underlying causes. If the causes are primarily subjective constructs then the implication must be that potentially so are the solutions. Surely, if coronary heart disease – or even more amazingly, shorter height – are caused by subjectively experienced low status then the solutions lie in improving status perceptions and not by, for example, providing better diets and accommodation and acting upon other social determinants.

The inequality theorists' focus on status has been critiqued. It is based on a series of underlying assumptions that are unlikely to be true in every case: for example, that income is a direct reflection of status differences; that status comparisons have more negative than positive effects – that is, that people compare themselves more critically to those above than positively to those below – and that this imbalance is more or less equal throughout the income inequality hierarchy. The approach assumes that status as a cause of health inequality operates in the same way across the status hierarchy, as opposed, for example, to lower-income groups being more influenced by financial problems while upper-income groups are more concerned with status. Given its subjective nature, status cannot be predicted to operate in the same way in different circumstances or with different people or groups. An example from my own research might serve to illustrate this. Having interviewed a man who had worked in a shoe factory all of his life I noticed he kept returning to one story of a colleague, whom he first described as a 'good chapel man', implying his colleague had a certain moral, and friendship status. However, when the colleague accepted the post of foreman in the shoe factory – a financial, hierarchical and status advance – outlooks changed. The action was interpreted by the interviewee, who was also the trade union representative in the factory, as a betrayal of class allegiance. These was a loss of status measured by the subjective opinions of the interviewee.[9] It is not possible to measure health impacts with such subjective tools. Status doesn't work in the constrained and focused ways that Marmot and other inequality theorists want it to. Studying Marmot's Whitehall materials provides obvious evidence that, though useful in a limited sense, comparing health outcomes in a specific workplace and using status as the yardstick with which to analyse health differences is not sufficient.

There is a problem with the linear progressions Marmot and other inequality theorists want to make. Marmot adopts a life course approach, using statistical analysis and drawing conclusions from averaging results. As the influential Marxist biologist Stephen Jay Gould points out, however, there is a danger with this set of techniques in producing, through the methodologies you use, results that do not fully – or at all – reflect and illustrate the variety and the non-linear developments involved in the processes being observed. As Gould puts it: 'There is a fallacy in reasoning about trends – a focus on particulars or abstractions … egregiously selected from a totality because we perceive these limited and uncharacteristic examples as moving somewhere – when we should be studying variation in the entire system and its changing pattern spread through time.'[10] In the case of the Whitehall studies, Gould's approach would require the researchers to look beyond the narrow constraints of workplace status to broader categories influencing health. While it is important to show that all elements of employment are likely to cause health-threatening stress and anxiety, including potentially subjective perceptions of status, it is important to investigate the 'entire system' informing health, which will include such social determinants of health as low pay, poor accommodation, poor diet and so on. The relationships described in the Whitehall studies in fact are not linear but dialectical, each informing the other in myriad interrelating ways inside and outside the employment context, each the cause and potential solution of the other.

Inequality theory has drawn on the work of Putnam and his concept of social cohesion/trust to try to explain differences in health outcomes between and within countries and communities. In a study of Italy, Putnam contends that northern Italy was more socially and econom-ically successful than southern Italy because the north had developed greater 'social capital', that is, more extensive social networks and greater social 'trust' than had the south.[11] Drawing on these findings, inequality theory argues that higher income inequality lowers social cohesion and lowers trust, which in turn produces poorer health outcomes. The inequality theorists' arguments have been critiqued on methodological grounds[12] and on the grounds of the vague notion of social cohesion by, among others, Professor of Public Health Sciences at the University of Toronto David Coburn.[13] Coburn elsewhere points out that inequality theory has in large part been devoted to attempts to explain how and why status is related to health. Wilkinson and Pickett's long anticipated follow-up book, *The Inner Level*, is a clear case in point. The focus here is on the psycho-social-biological mechanisms through which social factors are tied to health. Critics of their approach argue that not enough attention has been paid to the social, political and economic factors, and trends during the last quarter century that have contextualised the health-linked, psycho-social responses, as well as individuals' basic, physical well-being.[14] For Coburn, for example, the inequality theorists prefer to discuss general trends of health inequalities, mapping those on to psycho-social responses, rather than focusing on the material circum-stances of health inequality itself as discussed at length in Chapter 4. The issue of 'fat' poor people illustrates this.

Qualifying their contention that we now all wish to eat less, Wilkinson and Pickett describe the growing global concerns with obesity. They point to the 'major health crisis'[15] obesity represents and to the fact that both in the US and in the UK, levels of obesity, measured by body mass index, have rocketed, up from 15 per cent to 30 per cent between 1970 and today in the US and from under 10 per cent to over 25 per cent between 1980 and today in the UK. We know that obesity carries life-threatening health risks including hypertension, type 2 diabetes, cardiovascular disease, gallbladder disease and some cancers. The authors conclude, 'Trends in childhood obesity are now so serious that they are widely expected to lead to shorter life expectancies for today's children.'[16] As Chapter 4 described in some detail, the modern food industry, with a very small number of enormous food processing conglomerates controlling the quality of food globally, is failing to provide safe, nutritional and healthy food, especially for working-class and poorer working-class families and individuals. How our food supply is contextualised by this market-driven dietary commodity, produced for profit and not with health considerations primarily in mind, and how this affects our physical health, must surely be the starting point for any analysis of the obesity epidemic on health inequality generally. Disappointingly, however, Wilkinson and Pickett move on to consider the psycho-social impact of obesity, without giving sufficient consideration to the physicality of health affected by commodity food. They state that, 'Apart from the health consequences, obesity reduces emotional and social wellbeing.'[17] Research certainly supports this view, but instead of confronting the material forces and arguments framing the physical consequences of obesity, this trend channels discussion towards individualised solutions at the level of psychology, with which proponents of derisory public health initiatives like 'Eat five items of fruit a day' would be more than happy.

Coburn further develops his critique of the inequality theorists by analysing the effects of neoliberalism on health and class, with a specific focus on the issue of welfare cuts and their impact.[18] In a 2000 paper Coburn states:

Rather than income inequality producing lowered social cohesion and trust leading to lowered health status, neoliberalism (market dominance) produces both higher income inequality and lower social cohesion and presumably, either lowered health status or a health status which is not as high as it might otherwise have been. Neoliberalism has this effect partly through its undermining of particular types of welfare state.[19]

This is a global trend also affecting the Nordic countries previously lionised by inequality theory as more egalitarian and so less affected by inequality. In 2018, research by Rolf Aaberge and others concluded that European-wide policies of austerity had led to poorer sections of the region falling behind and health inequality growing as benefits and welfare provision cuts had an impact.[20] Even more interestingly, the report spells out what it regards as the material reasons underlying historically more equal health outcomes: 'A number of key institutions, notably collective bargaining, activation policies and wide access to high-quality education, reinforce each other, allowing a compressed wage distribution and extensive redistribution to co-exist with the high employment necessary to fund the extensive public services and transfers.'[21] The very empirical influences of strong trade unions and government funded and led education and welfare systems underpinned the relatively low rates of health inequality until these institutions were undermined as austerity measures began to bite. The Nordic example is particularly relevant as the area is identified by inequality theorists as an example of a region of egalitarianism likely to ensure better health in society as a whole. Clearly, as political contexts change and the Nordic region imposes austerity-driven cutbacks in welfare resources, health suffers – not as any reduction in status but as a result of, as Coburn argues, the policy and practice of neoliberalism 'undermining' social welfare.

Health is potentially undermined at a general level, through the impact of reductions in welfare provision on social determinants of health, like housing (having fewer social housing opportunities) diet (the declining quality and rising price of school meals) and the retreat from state provided healthcare systems towards ideas of health as a commodity. Research suggests that changes in UK welfare and benefits systems through the imposition of Universal Credit have increased the risk of ill health particularly, but not only, for potentially vulnerable groups such as disabled people, single parents and people leaving care institutions.[22] The introduction of Universal Credit in the UK has sparked a fresh rise in the number of sanctions – including on the sick and disabled, single parents and care leavers. In 2018, Frank Field, chairman of the Commons Work and Pensions Committee, said: 'We have heard stories of terrible and unnecessary hardship from people who've been sanctioned [by Universal Credit policy]. They were left bewildered and driven to despair at becoming, often with their children, the victims of a sanctions regime that is at times so counterproductive it just seems pointlessly cruel.'[23] In the US, research strongly suggests that poor welfare systems produce a 'mortality disadvantage'.[24] Jason Beckfield and Clare Bambra found evidence that 'the US mortality disadvantage is in part a welfare-state disadvantage'. They estimate that if the US had just the average standard of welfare provision of the other 17 OECD countries against which their research compared the US, the average life expectancy in the US would be approximately 3.77 years longer. As they conclude:

> The United States has a mortality disadvantage relative to its political and economic peer group. Previous research has focused on lifestyle and health care explanations. In this paper, we present the first long-term longitudinal examination of the contribution of the generosity of social policy programmes in explaining this disadvantage. Using life expectancy and indicators of unemployment insurance, pensions and sickness insurance, we found a substantively and statistically significant association between welfare generosity and population health especially in regards to pension provision. Our research suggests that there is evidence that the US mortality disadvantage is, in part, a welfare state disadvantage.[25]

For Coburn and others, understanding the material, social, political and economic causes of income inequality is key to understanding health inequalities, not individualised and subjectively experienced perceptions of status. To return to the example of the differences between north and south Italy, as used by Putnam, it was argued that differences in health outcomes between the two regions are based on the superior social cohesion and trust in the north. A report published in 2016 suggests a different picture. It found one in four Italians to be at risk of poverty, with the risk being almost twice as high in the south, seriously impacting their health expectations and outcomes.[26] Families with children are more at risk of poverty than at any time since records of this sort began.

It is estimated that a total of almost 17.5 million people live in poverty in Italy. Couples with at least three children face the highest risk, with 48.3 per cent of them struggling to make ends meet in 2015, up from 39.4 per cent the previous year. In the south, the rate of poverty in 2016 was 46.4 per cent, up from 2014. The situation was starkest in Sicily, where this figure rose to 55.4 per cent. This compares to 24 per cent in central Italy and 17.4 per cent in the prosperous north. Across Italy, half of families lived on an annual income of less than €24,190, a figure which fell to €20,000 in the south. The wealthiest 20 per cent of families took home more than 37 per cent of the total income, while the poorest 20 per cent accounted for just 7.7 per cent. 'From 2009 to 2014, salary in real terms has fallen for the poorest 20 per cent [increasing] the gap between the rich and poor.' The richest 20 per cent earned 4.9 times as much as the poorest when the report was published. A Save the Children report in 2015 said a third of Italian children were at risk of poverty, many of them living in cold or damp homes and missing out on educational and cultural opportunities with a clear and marked deterioration in their health as well as risks for their future health.[27]

Looked at this way, the economic impoverishment of southern Italy, due to specific political and historical developments, is the material cause of the poorer health outcomes of, at least some, of the population. Again, we must be wary of abstract generalisation and the 'fallacy in reasoning about trends' that premises all northern Italians as benefiting from better health than those in the south. The problem is a methodological and conceptual one. Putnam uses the limited and subjective concept of social cohesion as a means of analysis for trends and generalisations unsupported by material fact. This is not helpful at an academic or a practical level.

It is beyond doubt that the wealth of research and literature that has emerged over the last two decades detailing the extent to which health inequalities exist, and pointing to their links with income or wealth inequalities, has opened up the debate about the iniquitous nature of twenty-first-century global societies. A shortcoming of this 'inequality thesis', as this chapter has shown, lies in its use of subjective notions such as status, social cohesion and social trust, all of which are largely unmeasurable with any degree of accuracy or over time. This cannot provide a means of analysis or provide adequate solutions to the problems global populations face. Empirically based analysis of the broader categories included in the social determinants of health approach, dialectically applied in order to understand how each element impacts upon one another, can help us understand the root causes of health inequality and suggest ways of doing something about them.

6

Ageing Populations?

The concept of an ageing population, with its implicit reference to the idea that people are living longer, has particular relevance for a book on health and health inequality, since the average number of years that a person lives is one relatively crude measure of how healthy that population is. In a very real sense, it should be an occasion for celebration of a society's success. However, ageing population concepts are not usually thought of in this positive light. Most often, in science and popular discourse, the phrase conjures up images of global economies being burdened with an ever-increasing number of older people, living longer than ever and using up increasingly scarce healthcare resources while draining tax revenues by drawing on national pension pots for longer. Ageing population arguments have been called the 'voodoo demography' by their critics, a term first coined in 2000 in response to the growing clamour around the social costs associated with rising life expectancies.[1] So, while it is the case that the average ages of populations globally have increased over the last 20 years, including recently for those in many LMICs, there is an ideological element to the concept that needs to be understood. This chapter seeks to do that, in the process explaining how these averages are calculated, exploring the broader social factors underpinning the rise and arguing that people living longer is far from being a social negative.

Average life expectancies in the UK have increased consistently since the end of World War II. The number of people in their 70s in the UK increased from four million to five million between 1990 and 2016. Survival rates were far better for the post-World War II baby boom generation (born 1946 and onwards) than those born following the World War I baby boom (born 1920). Only 58 per cent of the 957,782 babies born in England and Wales in 1920 (turning 70 in 1990) survived to age 70, compared to 78 per cent of the 820,719 babies born in 1946 (turning 70 in 2016).[2] During this period a number of social and political developments coalesced to provide a general context highly supportive of good health. These elements include improvements in living conditions and diet, and the establishment of welfare provision, at the centre of which was the NHS. Coupled with these, the period from World War II through to the mid-1970s was one characterised by an extended period of high levels of full-time employment and job security and historically high rates of trade union membership. I will explain the relevance of trade union organisation to health and life expectancies in great detail in future chapters, but here I draw attention to the fact that the period of increased life expectancies which has resulted in an increase in the average age of the UK population coincides exactly with a period of growth in trade unions, reaching a peak of over 13 million in 1979.[3]

At the same time as we are witnessing the increased life expectancies of the so-called baby boomers, those born during the upsurge of birth rates for a 15-year period after World War II, there has been a falling away of birth rates from the late 1960s onwards. So, while the baby boom generations are living longer, birth rates are at historically low rates, producing the classic 'ageing population' profile.

However, concepts of ageing populations have become much more than descriptive categories and have taken on far-reaching ideological and political relevance, routinely being used to suggest that the globe is being swamped by hordes of older people using up scarce resources. Predictions abound, based on a continuing trend of ever-expanding life expectancies, that nations will not be able to cope so that both healthcare provision and pensions must be cut or limited. Let us first look at the idea that it is inevitable that life expectancies will continue to grow.

According to Marmot, research in 2017 strongly suggests that life expectancy growth in the UK has slowed or even stopped.[4] Using data from the Office for National Statistics, Marmot shows that the rate of increase in life expectancy has dropped by almost 50 per cent since 2010. Between 2000 and 2015, life expectancy at birth increased by one year every five years for women and by one year every 3.5 years for men. Post-2010, however, life expectancy for women has only increased by one year every ten years, with men's life expectancy increasing by one year every six years. Marmot says this shows that life expectancy growth has 'ground to a halt' after consistently rising over the past century. Marmot speculates that the past ten years of austerity are beginning to impact on life expectancies.[5] As Dorling points out, this decline is now recognised as the 'new norm'.[6]

We need to be clear from this point that although there has been a rise in life expectancies around the world, for many of the reasons I discuss below, life expectancies have remained unequally distributed in the consistency and extent of their growth. Life expectancy growth remains skewed by income such that those at the top end of income scales have enjoyed better health outcomes, including in terms of life expectancies. As I showed in Chapter 3, average life expectancies have been falling in the US for a decade and more. The top 10 per cent of income earners in the US continue to live longer than the rest, while at the bottom the last ten years have seen life expectancies for some – especially poor working-class women – actually decline. In the UK, Dorling's body of work is testimony to the class nature of health improvements including life expectancies. We need to bear this in mind as we work through the topic.

Marmot also suggests that 'remaining life expectancy' has slowed (in those aged 65 and over). Remaining life expectancy at age 65 is the average number of years people can expect to live past 65, which up until 2020 remains the retirement age in the UK for men. Remaining life expectancy had been increasing at a rate of one year every six years for women and one in every five for men. It has now significantly fallen to a one year increase every 16 years for women and every nine years for men.[7] A number of reasons are suggested for this, including a greater number of deaths attributed to dementia. Marmot points to the fact that dementia and Alzheimer's are regarded as the most common causes of death in women aged 80 and over (37,252 deaths) and in men aged 85 and over (12,258 deaths).[8] Dementia, its nature and its impact is a controversial topic, and I return to it later in this chapter.

Why did life expectancies increase so consistently in the years between the end of World War II and into the twenty-first century? Using a social determinant approach, we can begin to understand the rise in life expectancies through an historical analysis of some key social factors. Here I look at three of those already discussed: diet, housing and employment.

In the UK during and after World War II, governments took control of what people ate. The Ministry of Food was set up in 1939 to organise the provision of and to guarantee a nutritionally adequate diet for people during the war. It was the first organisation responsible for a nutrition policy in the UK. The ministry controlled all food supplies, food reserve stocks and distribution, and had local and regional committees to give expert information and organise the use of gardens, waste land and allotments for producing food locally. The ministry became a permanent department of state in 1946 until 1955, when it was subsumed within the Department for Agriculture and Fisheries to become the Ministry of Agriculture, Fisheries and Food. This was dissolved in 2002 and its responsibilities split between the Department for Environment, Food and Rural Affairs and the Food Standards Agency. As we can see, the state centrally planned and organised food supplies to ensure an adequate and equitable supply of food that properly nourished the UK population.

The National Food Survey (now known as the Family Food Survey) is the longest-running continuous survey of household food consumption and expenditure in the world. It was originally set up in 1940 by the Ministry of Food to monitor the adequacy of the diet of urban working-class households in wartime, and it was extended in 1950 to monitor households generally. It provides a wealth of information that has made a major contribution to the study of the changing patterns of household food consumption over time. During World War II, the British government introduced food rationing to make sure that everyone received their fair share of the limited food that was available. Food rationing started in 1940 and finally ended in 1954. To ensure good health, the amounts of available foods to cover people's nutrient needs were calculated using National Food Survey data. The wartime food shortages forced people to adopt new eating patterns. Most people ate less meat, fat, eggs and sugar than they had eaten before, but people with a poor diet previously, due to low incomes and poverty, were able to increase their intake of protein and vitamins.[9] Of course, being forced to ration food because of wartime shortage is not being suggested here as some kind of solution to the many food-related illnesses already discussed. But the fact remains that because food supplies were planned and disseminated centrally, under the control of a central authority basing their calculations on dietary need instead of profit, many people in the UK had a better diet during World War II than they had enjoyed before. This had a marked, and in some senses immediate effect on health outcomes. For example, infant mortality rates declined, and over time, as we have already seen, the average age at which people died from natural causes increased.[10]

Underpinning the general improvement in diet experienced by all and given great credit in terms of long-term health outcomes by research, is the support to children's diets provided by the state in the form of free school milk and cheap and nutritious school meals during and after World War II. Ellen Wilkinson, known as 'Red Ellen', was appointed the first woman minister of education by the post-war Labour government and oversaw the passage of the Free School Milk Act (1946). Wilkinson was from a working-class, socialist background, first coming to Parliament in 1924, actively supporting the general strike of 1926 and co-authoring a history of the strike, *The Workers' History of the Great Strike*, in 1927. She argued for the Labour Party to declare its support for Spanish forces opposing Franco in 1936, and in the same year helped organise the famous Jarrow March of unemployed workers from Jarrow to London. In 1947 she committed suicide, some arguing as a result of her deep disappointment at the underachievement of the post-war Labour government, with the Free School Milk Act her greatest achievement.[11] Free school milk for all, along with cheap and nutritious school meals, continued to be available for all school children for the next quarter of a century, and it is generally accepted that this was a key element of the increase in life expectancies over this period. Free school milk for all was ended in 1968 when the Labour government of Harold Wilson restricted it to junior school children only, and then to only those under seven years old by Secretary of State for Education Margaret Thatcher in 1971, when the first substantial increases in school meals were also sanctioned. We have yet to discover how this retreat from state intervention in children's diets will affect long-term health and life expectancies as the 1960s generations approach their sixties.

As with diet, the state played a key role in housing post-war. In the years following World War II the UK's housing stock was radically changed.[12] Between 1951 and 1960 the percentage of owner occupiers increased from 31 per cent to 44 per cent. Local authority renters rose from 17 per cent to 25 per cent while private renting fell from 52 per cent to 31 per cent as the state at national and local government level took the lead role in providing decent accommodation for post-war working people.[13] The Labour government of 1945–51 built just over a million homes as well as another half a million temporary houses, so-called 'Pre-Fabs' meant to provide temporary accommodation, many of which lasted for the next 30 years and more.[14] Several hundred thousand war-damaged properties were repaired as homelessness disappeared. The government intervened to keep rents low, capping them at 10 shillings per week. Tellingly, housing was placed under the control of the Ministry of Health, while the emphasis of the new homes was on housing of a decent size (at least three bedrooms, and a minimum of just over 80 square metres of space per housing unit) and good quality, to be a permanent, community resource.[15] The homes were for rent not for sale. Sociologist Piers Beirne describes post-war council housing as a 'temporary socialisation of money capital by Labour',[16] by which he means that building costs were determined outside of the profit nexus, as building and slum clearance were done by council staff who were directly employed at non-market rates. Local authorities were able to charge rents which reflected the cost of production of their housing stock rather than the going rates in the private rental market. Despite the fact that land ownership and the building industry remained in the hands of the private sector, as Beirne points out local and national government led the way, planning and providing safe and secure affordable housing for the next quarter of a century. Between 1951 and 1960 Conservative governments continued to build new homes, at the rate of 300,000 per year. This was more extensive house building than Labour had achieved, although the homes themselves were smaller: two bed rather than three bed and with a single upstairs toilet instead of the previous two. The minimum size was reduced to 750 square feet per building.[17] Tory Prime Minister Harold Macmillan himself boasted that his homes were 'quicker to build and cheaper to rent'. It is argued that part of the later dissatisfaction with council housing can be traced back to the worse quality of the homes built in the 1950s under Macmillan.[18]

By the mid-1960s much new-build housing took the form of high-rise concrete blocks. Buildings were designed in a modernist architectural style. The designers adopted as their models interwar European buildings such as Karl Marx House in Vienna.[19] For some planners, the tower blocks represented a positive change in the way people could live in increasingly crowded urban areas. One of the best known of the 1960s tower blocks is Balfron Tower, a 27-storey building at Rowlet Street in Poplar, east London. Designed by the Marxist architect Ernö Goldfinger, the tower was intended to give architectural expression to a vision of the city in which each year a smaller proportion of land space was available for housing. For Goldfinger, tower blocks freed up space for parks and children's playgrounds, improving the general environment in which people could live in more collective, community-based ways.[20]

As capitalism drifted past its post-war period of boom, housing, like other aspects of the social determinants of health, began to worsen, with the first substantial rent increases for council housing introduced by the Tories in the Housing Act of 1972, a slowdown in council house building and the move towards the sell-off of council housing during the 1980s. The degeneration of the tower block stock can also be rooted in this process of withdrawal of public funding for their upkeep. As with diet, governments withdrew from seeking to influence housing for the public good, leaving the reintroduced liberal market to determine building priorities, presaging a period of unparalleled housing shortage, price rise, rent rise and declining living space and general housing quality since then.

Chapter 10 discusses in detail how trade unions grew and strengthened during World War II, and explains how this fundamentally and positively impacted on health provision and health generally. Post-war, union officials and activists were keen to build on these successes. Many unions acknowledged and sought to take advantage of the new conditions in post-war Britain and looked for ways to adapt union organisation to them. Unions sought to become more inclusive in recognition of the nature and needs of the new workforce.

Employment in manufacturing had risen to an all-time peak of 39 per cent in 1951, and it remained at high levels throughout the decade.[21] Facing chronic labour shortages, employers began to adapt working conditions to attract women with childcare responsibilities back into work. Unions ran recruiting campaigns targeting women and created new internal structures to ensure women's voices could be heard and were reflected in union policy. As a result, the historically high level of 25 per cent of women employed in unions, reached in 1945, was maintained.[22] Union officials and activists made efforts to interest young people in unions and involve them in union activity. The trade union movement maintained some of the combative elements it had shown during war. Following a sharp recession in 1956 the British Motor Corporation made 6,000 workers at its Longbridge factory in Birmingham redundant without either pay or notice. The shop stewards' committee of the Amalgamated Engineering Union (AEU) called a strike, lasting for six weeks and actively supported by other car manufacture unions. In March 1957, national strikes in shipbuilding and engineering produced what the *Observer* described as 'the most serious crisis since 1926'[23] in industrial relations. The government successfully applied strong pressure on the employers to concede substantial wage increases. The AEU emerged with a renewed reputation for militancy and an increased membership. Young workers who had hitherto taken little interest in union affairs were drawn more deeply into the union through successful strike action, with many going on to form the backbone of trade union structures into the 1970s.[24] This continued post-war combativity and organisation ensured that this key social determinant of health – employment – is likely to have maintained its positive influence in general through to the late 1970s.

Using this social determinant of health approach, ageing populations can be seen as resulting from this combination of improvements in social aspects underpinning health – like diet, housing, employment, healthcare and social welfare – importantly guided and heavily influenced by the state intervening in these key areas. It can be argued that the increased life expectancies over the last 70 years have resulted from centrally planned, state-led provision across a range of health determinants. People living longer is a success story for the central planning, welfare enabled model, supported by strong working-class organisation through big and active trade unions.

It may be that the decline in life expectancies noted by Marmot is not primarily to do with austerity alone, but is contextualised by a more long-term move away from state responsibility for key aspects of people's socially determined health from the 1970s onwards. Time will tell.

Arguments first developed in the 1980s, initially by a group of right-wing American academics, seek to paint the success of increased life expectancy as the 'ticking time bomb' of overpopulation. The idea that there are more older people draining social resources has become a powerful political tool. The idea that population ageing is a bad thing originated in the US. It was informed by political, academic and popular media discourse. In 1984 Samuel Preston, at the annual Population Association of America, alluded to growing tensions between older and younger people. Preston claimed the young were the ones footing the bill for the rising healthcare costs associated with illness and disability related to old age.[25] Laurence Kotlikoff developed a 'generational accounting framework' using poorly evidenced data and assertions to develop a political argument for reform of social and economic policy to discredit and constrain older people's access to resources.[26]

Daniel Callahan remains a central proponent of ageing population ideologies. He argues that the ageing population is such a threat that healthcare and other welfare services for older people should be rationed and/or withheld from them. Callahan spent the 1960s editing *Commonweal*, a Catholic opinion journal, becoming an influential writer and author in Catholic intellectual circles. In addition to articles in *Commonweal* he wrote or edited nine books, including *Honesty in the Church* and *The Catholic Case for Contraception*. In 1987, Callahan published his most influential book, *Setting Limits: Medical Goals in an Aging Society*, which argued that US society would need to limit expensive care for older Americans. The *New York Times Book Review* wrote at the time: 'This is a pivotal work that poses hard questions and proposes provocative answers. *Setting Limits* promises to be the benchmark for future moral, medical and policy discussions of aging.'[27] The book was controversial from the start. A major critique was developed by Barry and Bradley exposing Callahan's underlying views that beyond a certain age death, not life, serves the true interests of older people.[28] As they show, this repugnant and deeply hypocritical view provides ideological cover for those political interests which seek to reduce healthcare and welfare provision, as expressed by Reagan and Thatcher and since then. Given that Ronald Reagan was 78 as Callahan wrote, we can safely assume that Callahan didn't include him in his death-not-life philosophy.

The critique of what has become known as Callahan's and others' 'voodoo demography' points to the many flaws in ageing population concepts, their almost complete lack of evidence base and the numerous and fundamental methodological flaws. At a methodological level, one of the key problems is the use of dependency ratios as a measure of the costs of changing social age structures. The dependency ratio is an age-population ratio of those not in the labour force (the dependent parts are the ages 0–14 and 65+) and those typically in the labour force (the productive part, ages 15–64). The method makes claims to provide an estimate of the extent of the productive population. With the changing pensionable ages and the growth of older people remaining in work past retirement ages, the concept is, in practice, becoming less and less reliable.[29]

Demographers Ellen Gee and Gloria Gutman show that defining everyone over 65 as dependent on social support and on others in society is completely arbitrary, homogenises older people's experiences and removes their contribution from the equation.[30] Jeroen Spijker and John MacInnes argue that in the UK, as in North America, the old-age dependency ratio defines all people above the statutory pension age as dependent, regardless of their economic, social or medical circumstances. The authors show that, with a simple adjustment of this ratio to take into account projected life expectancies and the numbers of people in employment, far from rising, dependency levels over the last four decades have actually fallen. This completely undermines the politico-ideological case for restructuring healthcare and welfare provision. As they point out, regarding older people's levels of dependency:

> Over one million are still working, mostly part time, many with valuable experience or specialist knowledge. The spending power of the 'grey pound' has risen inexorably. Many do volunteer work vital to the third sector or look after grandchildren. We know that most acute medical care costs occur in the final months of life, with the age at which these months occur having little [economic] effect.[31]

Far from being a burden, older people continue to contribute to society in a huge variety of ways. For example, as a result of spiralling childcare costs, hundreds of thousands of families all over the UK depend on grandparents to look after children while parents work. In 2018, the vast majority of grandparents failed to claim government benefits for doing this, saving the government millions.[32]

At an economic level, and underpinning ageing population concepts, is the idea that globally (predominantly in the highly industrialised economies) populations have grown to such an extent that governments can no longer afford to pay decent pensions or sustain traditional retirement ages. In the UK and across Europe governments over the last decade and more have sought to reduce pension payments and increase the age of retirement.[33]

For critics of the government pensions agenda, sitting alongside voodoo demography is the 'pensions myth'.[34] The idea is that because people are living longer global economies can no longer sustain traditional retirement ages. Existing pension arrangements are no longer feasible and must be changed, goes the argument. This approach is predicated on the idea that resources are finite and strictly limited, that pensions can only be drawn from a specific social care pot and that other areas of state spending, such as military spending, cannot be touched. The argument does not stand up to scrutiny. There is no reason, apart from political choice, why funds from a range of other spending areas funded through taxation could not be used to fund pensions. For example, governments could raise more revenue with a more effective and fairer tax system. It is now well established that, through tax evasion (illegal) and tax avoidance (legal), Britain's capitalist sector is not paying up to £70 billion a year in tax that they ought to. Ending offshore schemes, accountancy tricks and downright fraud could deliver 4–5 per cent of GDP in extra revenue and thus easily cover the so-called pensions gap. It could even go on to provide a far more adequate pension. A more progressive tax system that taxed the rich more and poor people less would yield more revenue.[35]

In 2018, the UK government spent 3 per cent of GDP on military spending to fund its global military interventions. It wastes billions annually on procurement of military equipment, averaging £36 billion annually between 2013 and 2019.[36] Governments are happy to spend tax money on business incentives and subsidies, tax relief on private education and £37 billion a year on private pensions (better used for state pensions). The 2008 bailout of the banking system in the UK accounted for 10 per cent of GDP. A redistribution of government spending plus an increase in government revenues, without taxing the average household one penny more, is perfectly possible and would easily yield the extra funds required to raise the state pension as well as providing the potential to increase other services.[37]

Pensions right across Europe have consistently been a target of government action, with national governments using varieties of ageing population arguments to justify this. But the real cause of the so-called pensions crisis was the economic crash of 2008, not too many older people. 'Rapid policy' changes[38] following the financial crash saw immediate pensions reductions for older people in Greece, Hungary, Ireland, Italy, Latvia, Portugal, Romania and Spain.[39] It is important to note that resistance to cuts in pensions has been common and has often led to governments backing away from fully implementing plans.[40]

In the UK change has been slower but nonetheless substantial. The UK economy grows at about 2.25 per cent a year on average (after taking into

account booms and slumps). On the basis of this general trend, governments have argued that the current state pension cannot be maintained.
State pensions set to be available to men and women at age 66 by the
year 2020, in 2017 cost about £71 billion in real terms, or 4.7 per cent
of UK GDP.[41] On the current estimates of the increase in the number of
state pensioner units (as it is called to include married couples) from 8.5
million now to 11.5 million by the end of the decade, the cost will rise
in real terms to £89 billion, or 5.1 per cent of GDP, while the average
weekly value of that pension will fall from £160 a week to £148 per week.
Paying for the state pension will rise and the value of that pension to each
pensioner will fall in real terms (after inflation). However, if the economy
grew by just 1 per cent more the situation is utterly different. Now real
GDP rises as fast as the number of pensioners grows, and the burden on
the economy actually falls from 4.7 per cent of GDP (in 2010 terms) to
4.3 per cent, while the real value of the weekly state pension rises from
£160 a week to £164 a week.[42] The increased number of pensioners could
be catered for without any change in the share of spending going to the
state pension and with even a small increase in the real value of that
pension. If an economy grows fast enough or, better, if more of the total
value of what is produced year on year by working people was realised as
socialised value rather than being syphoned out of the system as private
profit, we already generate enough wealth to be able to support older
people.

In the UK, the replacement rate (the ratio of the state pension to
average earnings) is one of the lowest in the OECD, just 33 per cent
in 2010 (compared to an average 50 per cent in the richer capitalist
economies).[43] That means that the average pensioner with just a state
pension must live on one-third of what they were earning on average
at work. This has already led to a steep rise in pensioner poverty. The
Joseph Rowntree Foundation warned in 2018 that one in six pensioners
is now living in poverty as a result of derisory state pensions, soaring
rents and an austerity-driven benefits freeze. Pensioner poverty is rising,
meaning that many are having to choose between paying for heating and
buying food each winter. A further one in three UK pensioners are 'at
risk of poverty' compared with just 19 per cent for the EU average. By
2016–17, 16 per cent of pensioners were living in poverty, rising to 31
per cent among those in social housing and 36 per cent among private
renters.[44] The UK spends just 5.7 per cent of GDP on pensions (state,

public and private) compared with 7.2 per cent average in the OECD. Yet, in the UK, we have 27 per cent of our working population aged over 65 compared to 24 per cent in the OECD. Britain's pensioners have the fourth highest level of poverty in Europe, worse off even than Romanian and Polish pensioners in relative poverty terms.[45] This is a key element of ageing population arguments in the UK. Instead of explaining the worsening living conditions of older people in terms of systematic failings of capitalism and the political choices made by governments on behalf of the employing class, older people themselves are blamed for being a burden on declining welfare resources and for having the temerity to still be alive. As in the 1800s, when Malthusian-inspired social commentators blamed the so-called high fertility rates of poor people for using up social resources, the ageing population argument puts the blame on too many older people for the poverty they experience.

Evidence clearly shows that the most efficient way of delivering a decent pension for all would be to fund all pensions totally from taxation and other government revenues and administer it through a government pension agency. It would be the most equitable, cheapest to run and simple to understand. Even the Turner report on UK pensions, commissioned by the then Labour government in 2009, admitted that the cheapest, most equitable and effective pension scheme would be a universal taxation-funded state pension for all without means testing and doing away with costly private pension fund managers. The government's own report shows that a centrally planned, funded and administered system would be vastly superior to the market-driven ad hoc schemes currently being touted.[46]

The financial crisis of 2008 and what has been called the 'Long Depression' that has followed[47] is the main cause of the growing deficits in public (and private) pension schemes. The financial collapse has led to losses or lower returns in private sector 'funded' schemes that are invested heavily in the stock market. Of the UK's 'funded' private pension schemes, 60 per cent are invested in the stock market compared with only 36 per cent in the OECD average. Funded schemes returns depend on the vagaries of the stock and bond markets. By 2011, according to the Pension Protection Fund, private sector pension fund assets covered only 83 per cent of the potential payouts because of the falls in global stock markets.[48] A survey by the UK's Confederation of British Industry found that in 2017, 71 per cent of employers thought their company pension schemes were 'under water'.[49] This is not because too many people needed them but because of poorly performing stocks and shares.

The pensions myth is just that. Decent pensions for all is not impossible or unaffordable, even during a period of rising populations. They are a matter of political choice, not numbers of people.

The medicalisation of the ageing process is a widely discussed topic. Senility was long thought of as inevitable in old age, until the 1980s when public awareness of dementia grew and funds for dementia research dramatically increased. Since then, dementia has not been considered a natural phenomenon of ageing but has become a medical problem with biological causes and subject to drug treatment. Through the process of biomedicalisation, senility, which has been considered appropriate to age, is now 'a deviance, a medical problem and a clinical entity with distinct pathology and requiring specific treatment'. As a result, all coexisting symptoms or illnesses, such as depression, have been brought in under the umbrella of dementia, regardless of whether they may simply reflect a normal emotional response to a deteriorating social context. All features that come along with dementia tend to be seen as part of the constellation of symptoms and signs in dementia or an indicator of a disease stage. Fears of the costs involved in sustaining expanding older populations are further deepened through reference to rising healthcare costs associated with specific age-related illness, particularly dementia. The so-called 'dementia epidemic' comes with its own constructions of older people as costly burdens, with predictions of the exponential growth of demented older people draining the public coffers and claiming millions in dementia research to find a drug-related 'cure'. Again, this needs careful inspection.

Carol Brayne of Cambridge University and chair of the Cambridge Institute for Public Health and various other academic and policy-framing bodies questions the perceived wisdom with regard to dementia worries. Brayne and her colleagues have developed a critique of dementia and Alzheimer's disease, based on a series of in-depth longitudinal studies.[50] She argues that people 'tend to talk about dementia as if it's a disease that you have or you haven't'.[51] In fact, dementia is a syndrome that impairs the mental function of earlier life and which can interfere with daily activities. Her arguments suggest that any impact of dementia is dependent on the culture and society you live in: 'If you live in a society where elders are supported within households with multiple generations and few demands are placed on older individuals, decline due to dementia can be substantial before it is seen as a problem.'[52] In other words, dementia is culturally relative, it's impact limited or increased according to the nature of society in which you live. The exact causes of dementia are not known and may be too complex ever to fully comprehend. However, research suggests that key risk factors include diabetes, stroke, midlife obesity, midlife hypertension, depression, smoking, low education and low physical activity. As Brayne and others point out, these factors are clearly associated with wealth inequalities or, more simply, class. As we have already seen, diabetes, obesity, hypertension, depression and more are socially determined illnesses associated with low-income groups. As Brayne argues, the evidence shows that social deprivation is likely to increase the risk of dementia. Brayne found that contrary to numerous predictions of dementia epidemics, the estimated number of people with dementia has remained relatively stable over time. This is despite a substantial increase in the proportion of the population in the oldest age groups. This amounted to a proportionate fall in dementia rates. Drawing on social determinant themes Brayne concludes: 'This population has lived through the period after the Second World War, when a socialized health and welfare system was introduced, reducing inequalities. Education was more widely available, child health improved, including immunization and access to healthcare, and people were better nourished. All of this resulted in people living longer in better health at old ages.'[53]

The cultural relativity approach is powerfully supported by studies from South East Asia which show that nearly half of dementia patients surveyed had no complaints about cognitive function three years before diagnosis, suggesting that there is a discrepancy between objective cognitive impairment identified by tests and subjective functional impairment in daily life. Research concluded that 'environmental support' and 'cultural relativism', were key in understanding these discrepancies.[54]

Research shows that early stage dementia sufferers retain insight about their condition and develop adaptive behaviours. Families play an important role in this. The extended family remains, conceptually, the basic family unit in many Asian societies, although the nuclear family is becoming dominant. Extended families mean daily lives are less affected by mild cognitive dysfunctions such as memory impairment since meals, transportation, health and so on can be taken care of by family members.

People are not considered diseased until the late stage of dementia, for example, when they no longer recognise people. In societies constructed around the nuclear family even mild cognitive impairment can severely effect abilities to cope. For example, in areas with poor public transport systems driving skills are a basic requisite to mobility. Loss of the ability to get around by yourself means a loss of independence and potentially accelerated cognitive decline. This is less of a problem for older people who live in a more self-contained community with no need to drive on their own. In other words, dementia is likely to impact less in more collectivised, mutually supportive environments.[55]

In a society which values independent responsibility and reward as a social norm, even mild impairment in cognitive performance can reduce individual abilities to perform daily activities. In societies based on individualism, ones governed by a curative approach to healthcare and the medicalisation of an expanding range of human behaviours, those who come to regard themselves as having non-normal health patterns will ask a doctor for a diagnosis. Any perceived decline in cognitive ability may become associated with a specific, medical diagnosis. In different – historical and geographical – cultures, forgetfulness has been regarded as part of the ageing process, just as we do not expect older people to move as fast as younger people.[56] In some cultures, cognitive impairment may be conceptualised, studied and experienced in a totally different way from the ageing processes. For example, in 'no ageing in India', dementia is understood not as an individual health condition but seen as a metaphor for the moral decay of the family and nation.[57]

An ageing population is a description of a period of historic growth in the age of global populations due to specific historical reasons, as explained above, most notably as a result of the centralised control of key social determinants of health for an extended period following World War II. More often, concepts of ageing populations are used in ideological-political ways to construct older people as a social burden: a drain on economic and healthcare resources. This chapter has shown that this is not the case. It has shown that ageing population arguments seek to blame 'too many old people' for the decline in social care resources available to them and the conditions of poverty in which an increasing proportion of them live. This reduction in resources is actually rooted in the political choices of the governing class. The chapter has shown that the idea that modern societies cannot afford proper pensions and provision for older people is a myth and that any current pensions 'crisis' is rooted in systemic failures of boom and bust capitalism. It has shown there is no dementia epidemic and that this is a culturally relative syndrome, not a disease, and a diagnosis overused for political ends as old age becomes increasingly medicalised.

An alternative view of this historically specific shift in the average age of global populations is to see older people as a resource that we as a society can choose to cherish, use and subsequently support. Not only have the over 70s contributed to the historically exceptional levels of wealth created since the end of World War II, they possess skills, knowledge and experiences from which younger generations can learn. The over 70s are an assimilation of the collective learning and knowledge creation of the twentieth century and should be acknowledged and celebrated as such. That they aren't is a consequence of political choice made by the employing class which, if it remains unchallenged, endangers the future longevity and health of the rest of us.

7

Health, Power and Paradigms

There are all sorts of positive things about the influence of people like Foucault and Derrida, we're clearly in their debt in lots of ways ... in terms of the reaction against post-structuralism that we've seen over the last ten or fifteen years [it is] because of their principle rejection of totalization. I mean, to put it simplistically, what's missing from all of their discourses is capitalism.[1]

This chapter looks at ways of theorising how modern concepts of something called 'health' arose historically across Europe and beyond. It begins by looking at the work of Michel Foucault, whose work has had a major impact on health studies over the course of the twenty-first century. I compare and contrast the post-structuralist approach of Foucault to the more empirical stance taken by Alfons Labisch, a leading European sociologist. I develop a comparative analysis of the social and political roles the medical profession plays in the twenty-first century. Further, and drawing on the work of the philosopher of science Thomas Kuhn, considering why, at particular points in history, medical roles and the ideas underpinning them have radically changed. I shine a spotlight on the relationship between doctors as social actors, the development of the scientific and professional skills they possess and how and why these change in the context of broader social forces. The chapter takes its lead from Foucault's third major work, *The Birth of the Clinic*, published in 1963, in which he first develops his notion of what has become known as the 'medical gaze' in a broader analysis of the effects the French Revolution had on health, healthcare practice and health studies.

It is not possible to overstate the extent to which the French Revolution of 1789 affected the ideas, science and practice of healthcare and our understanding of health. Wholesale reforms of medical policies and institutions were enacted. New programmes of medical inquiry, new disease concepts and new research practices were introduced. Post-revolutionary governments took control of hospitals and other health provision away from the church. As a result, in revolutionary France medicine was 'characterised by scientific observation and raised on pathological anatomy'.[2] As the philosopher-doctor Pierre Cabanis put it, post-revolutionary France's golden rule became 'read little, see much, do much'.[3]

The Birth of the Clinic considers issues to do with disease, health and health services that arose in popular debate during the eighteenth and nineteenth century as part of Foucault's analysis of power and relations of power in society then and now. In the course of this he develops a critique of what he regards as some of the myths of the French Revolution's impact on modern concepts of health and health services. Central to his critique is his discussion of the debate around hospitals. Throughout this period, before, during and after the revolution hospitals in France were criticised as 'temples of death', more akin to the UK workhouses of the nineteenth century. For example, in 1772 Dr Jean Gilibert of the Faculté at Montpellier wrote a three-volume work entitled Anarchy – or Medicine Considered as an Evil in Society[4] describing some of the inadequacies of hospital provision and the lack of expertise of doctors. Bertrand Barère de Vieuzac, who presided over the trial that led to the execution of Louis XVI in 1793, proclaimed that an aim of the revolution must be 'No more poorhouses, no more hospitals'.[5] The radical faction of the revolution – the Mountain, led by Robespierre and Danton – demanded the abolition of hospitals, regarding them as an institutionalisation of poverty. Gustave Le Bon asked, 'Must any section of mankind be sick and needy ... Therefore let notices be placed over the gates of these asylums announcing their coming disappearance. For if when the revolution is complete we still have such unfortunates amongst us our revolutionary work will have been in vain.'[6] When the Mountain briefly took power in 1793–4, the idea of an organisation of public assistance by governments and of the abolition of the old hospitals was in principle accepted.

The constitution of 1793 in its Declaration of Rights states that 'public assistance is a sacred debt'; the law statutes drawn up later that year ordered the creation of a 'great book of national beneficence' and the organisation of a system of state assistance throughout the countryside. Provision was made for 'houses of health' for 'the sick who have no home or who cannot receive help there'.[7] In this way, the most radical edge of the French Revolution for the first time in history joined together the question of poverty and ill health and argued for state assistance to avoid both, declaring the hospital system as 'an anachronistic solution that does not respond to the real needs of the poor and that stigmatises the sick in a state of penury'.[8] In their place the revolutionaries argued for, in embryo, an interlinking system of outreach doctors employed by the state supported by nationwide health centres, proposing a fundamental shift away from the old hospitals.

The Revolution took control of health provision away from traditional health hierarchies, setting up the Société Royale de Médecine which usurped the previously dominant Faculté with its roots in feudalism. The Société was tasked with linking 'French medicine with foreign medicine by means of a useful correspondence; to gather together isolated observations, to preserve them and to compare them; and above all to research into the causes of common diseases, to forecast their occurrence and to discover the most effective remedies for them'.[9] As Foucault points out, with this aim set for them the French medical profession became the 'collective consciousness of pathological phenomena', a development which Foucault rather dismissively ascribes to the 'novelty value' of the revolutionary process.[10] Here, Foucault at best understates the extent to which the shift in ways of studying and practising medicine, implicit in this measure, changes the path along which medicine – in France and elsewhere as a consequence – developed from this point on. In brief, as Kuhn puts it, a paradigm shift in medicine occurred as a result of the socio-political changes in French society generally, a point to which I return. Medicine stopped being the concern of a few learned men, breaking the back of the traditional medical hierarchies, and became the concern of the state, with responsibilities and a determination to include the population at large in health research and practice. From the beginning of the revolution there were calls for research to be decided by democratically elected commissions of state-employed doctors, and that 'government health centres' should be created in every major town and a 'health court' established in Paris, sitting alongside the National Assembly, coordinating the health research and health reform projects enacted in the following years, with powers to distribute resources around the country.[11]

Similarly, a preventative model of health began to evolve. A report by Lespagnol in 1790 highlighted the shortage of practitioners in rural areas. As a result, new solutions emerged. These included the duty of rural doctors to collect and collate important medical information, like family histories of disease, but also including reflections on social determinants of health which might be at play – like observations about the topography and weather in specific regions, the housing people lived in, the work that people did and so on. As well as collecting information, as part of the collective consciousness of the nation's health doctors had a responsibility to 'supplement his supervisory activity with teaching, for the best way of avoiding the propagation of disease is to spread medical knowledge'.[12] In other words, over a few years, as a consequence of revolutionary upheaval, in principle the reign of the old hospitals was ended and movements towards their closure begun, health research and practice was collectivised and centred on an outreach-based state-employed medical profession, the old medical order was overturned, the principal of a service based around health centres was accepted and a preventative model of health set in train, expressing at least the potential for a 'generalised medical consciousness, diffused in space and time, open and mobile, linked to each individual existence as well as to the collective life of the nation'.[13]

Given all of this, it is unfortunate that Foucault seems largely disparaging of this progress in thought, instead using much of this to develop the concept of the medical gaze. The medical gaze is a way of seeing that involves the physician in a 'double system of observation' – one that discovers the disease process and 'circumscribes its natural truth'.[14] Under it a person's 'constitution' is a collective of bodily interrelationships that can be interpreted only by a physician. Facts about the body are determined by the physician's medical gaze – his sensations, perceptions, experiences and so on – rather than having an independent existence to be discovered and analysed. Foucault argues that the gaze is also an ideological tool:

There is a spontaneous and deeply rooted convergence between the requirements of political ideology and those of medical technology. In a concerted effort, doctors and statesmen demand ... the suppression of every obstacle to the constitution of this new [ideological] space ... Liberty is the vital, unfettered force of truth. It must therefore have a world in which the gaze, free of all obstacle, is no longer subjected to the immediate law of truth: the gaze is not faithful to truth, nor subject to it, without asserting, at the same time, a supreme mastery: the gaze that sees is the gaze that dominates.[15]

Looked at through this lens, many of the issues discussed above become merely adaptations of systems of health in order to facilitate greater levels of social control. For example, the collection of health data from localities becomes a way for the state to keep watch over its citizenship, described by Foucault as facilitating a 'generalised presence of doctors whose intersecting gazes form a network and exercise at every point in space, and at every moment in time, a constant, mobile, differentiated supervision'.[16] This, rather sinister, interpretation of the doctor's role evolving during this period of social and political upheaval is both one-dimensional and historically decontextualised. It seeks to locate ideological power in the medical profession itself, with doctors sharing as equals, rather than being subject to, the political interests of the dominant political class, securing ideological hegemony over the populace in their own interests.

This view is challenged by Alfons Labisch in his paper 'The Social Construction of Health'.[17] Labisch explores the development of a modern German working class in the latter part of the nineteenth and early twentieth centuries through an analysis of 'change from extensive to intensive use of labour: instead of short-term exhaustion of the proletariat [industrial working class] by work, it became necessary to secure permanently a labour reserve of sufficient quality and numbers'.[18] Specifically, Labisch analyses the development of industrial capitalism in Germany from the 1870s to investigate how the concept of 'health' was historically constructed as an ideological tool with which the German employing class developed the workforce it needed. The author explains how this was used to shape the attitudes and behaviours of the workforce. Health concepts gave structure to the change from a workforce based on the rapid turnover of semi-skilled labour through work exhaustion (something Labisch calls the 'Manchester School' approach after the model used by employers during the early history of industrialisation in the UK) to one based on a relatively 'healthy' – that is to say, one still able to work – workforce sustainable over time.[19]

As with the growth of the UK proletariat from the 1780s onwards, to the Chinese proletariat of the twenty-first century, the German urban working class first took shape through rural workers moving to industries based in and around growing urban areas. In the process of this – and in common with any mass movement of populations from rural to urban areas – traditional support systems, community life and patterns of behaviour break down or become inappropriate to the new constraints of urban living and working. The employing class needed behaviours to be 'complemented and replaced by artificial and institutional equivalents' in order that the newly urbanised populations could be 'colonized and assimilated'[20] into the new demands of urban-based industrialisation. Labisch argues that, in the German context, a medicalised version of a concept of health became central to this process. The concept carries with it numerous advantages as an ideological tool. 'Health' is presented as a scientifically definable and personally attainable goal, neutral and free from ideological agendas.[21]

In the emergent world of industrial capitalism, where the proletariat owned nothing but her or his labour to sell, health becomes central. Without it, there is no possibility of work and no survival so that, Labisch argues, health becomes 'life's supreme goal' and the worker 'subordinates his manner of life entirely to principles of health derived from medicine'.[22] The process is facilitated by the medical profession, establishing its monopoly over medical practice. Implicit in this process of medical monopoly is the suppression of folk medicine, lay healers (quacks) and traditional interpretations of health.[23] (As a footnote, it's interesting to compare Foucault's treatment of 'quacks', whom the arch critic of professional medicine regards as dangerous charlatans – some undoubtedly were – with Labisch, who regards 'quacks' as traditional sources of medical advice and help suppressed by the developing European medical hierarchies.) As Labisch concludes: 'In this professional medical monopoly context, the ideological concept "health" could be "politically channelled, individualised and made into a therapeutic problem … an instrument both for a neutral controlling of behaviour and for a socially pacificatory way of dealing with social problems".'[24]

In his *Limits to Medicine*, Ivan Illich develops this question of medical monopoly further in his analysis of 'radical monopoly':

Ordinary monopolies corner the market; radical monopolies disable people from doing or making things on their own … They impose a society-wide substitution of commodities for use-values by reshaping the milieu and by appropriating those of its general characteristics which have enabled people so far to cope on their own … The malignant spread of medicine … turns mutual care and self-medication into misdemeanours or felonies.[25]

Health ideologies embedded in medicalised practice and systems of governance become disabling and controlling, laying down behavioural pathways for us to follow and of primary benefit to the employing class. For Labisch, Illich and others, health ideologies are deeply rooted in the material needs of capitalist profit.

Though both Foucault and Labisch want to examine the influence the medical profession has over behaviour, each sites this influence in different, sociological spaces. For Foucault, the 'medical gaze' is how doctors exert their professional power which 'converges' with the ideological needs of the employing class. For Labisch, ideological power is located not directly in the medical profession but in concepts of 'health', to which doctors themselves are also subject. Even though doctors may mostly unconsciously contribute to the ideological power of the health concept – through medical roles, institutions and popular beliefs – the concept has evolved to serve, not the needs of doctors themselves, but the needs of an employing class.

It is a matter of fact that sitting at a desk and staring at a computer screen for eight or more hours every day is unhealthy. As a recent NHS survey states: 'Studies have linked excessive sitting with being overweight and obese, type 2 diabetes, some types of cancer, and early death. Sitting for long periods is thought to slow the metabolism, which affects the body's ability to regulate blood sugar, blood pressure and break down body fat.'[26] It is also a fact that over the last 20 years more and more of us earn our living by doing this. It is undoubtedly the case that your local GP knows it's unhealthy. Perhaps you will have been to your doctor with a bad back, or bad neck or wrist or lower arm problems, or indeed worries that you might have diabetes. Has any reader ever had his doctor prescribe 'two weeks not sitting at your desk working'? It is unlikely, because this is not within the remit of the health dialogue doctors are presented with by the accepted notions of 'health' they are tasked with protecting and disseminating. Doctors are in an ideological cleft stick and the extent to which they are aware of this is a measure of how aware they are of their own lack of opportunity to propose meaningful, health-giving solutions. The situation carries with it mental health risks, and suicide rates for doctors are climbing. For example, in the UK between 2011 and 2015 430 doctors committed suicide.[27] In the US, between 300 and 400 doctors commit suicide each year, the highest among the so-called 'professional occupations' category.[28]

The internal conflict and frustration arising from the contradictory social position of doctors – driven by a desire to help, frustrated from doing so by the constraints of accepted and ideological notions of 'health' by which they must largely abide – bubbled to the surface in the UK during the junior doctors' strikes of 2016 and 2017. The strikes began in January of 2016 after 98 per cent of the nearly 38,000 junior doctors who took part in the strike ballot voted for strike action, the first such action in over 40 years. Much of the commentary around both phases of the strike, in the first instance caused by the then Conservative government's insistence on forcing new contracts of employment on junior doctors, pointed to the fact that doctors felt that this attack on their pay and conditions endangered their own well-being in the job, as well as the safety of patients.[29] Doctors complained of the pay cuts implicit in the new contracts and having to 'live from one pay cheque to another', with the consequence of having to do extra work on weekend and evening rotas.[30] There was a fall in morale and diminished loyalty to the NHS leading up to the strike: 'Attitudes of doctors have changed – where does the loyalty lie if we are not being treated fairly?' a doctor asked.[31] There was a perception of more doctors leaving the UK to work abroad, and a sense of a falling number of doctors being left behind to carry the increasingly unbearable load. The strikes ended but the narrative behind them continues to evolve.

This does not look like an empowered clique, exercising their power through a 'medical gaze'. It looks like a group of highly skilled workers alienated from their labour. Here is not the place to engage in a long discussion about the nature of alienation, a concept that has made its way through history and found itself in its final formulation to date in the hands of Karl Marx and later Marxists. Suffice to say, in essence alienation is having something taken away from you. For example, the Punjab Land Alienation Act of 1900 was a piece of legislation passed by the British Raj that took away land from indigenous ownership. In a capitalist society, in order to survive we are forced to sell the only thing we have, our ability to work. For Marxists work fundamentally defines us as human beings. When we sell our labour we are in effect parting with part of what makes us human. Our human potential is diminished because we do not get back – in wages – what we give in labour. When we sell our labour and the products of our labour they become commodities. What do doctors produce? We might agree that along with other healthcare workers they use their knowledge and practical skills to produce care or, strictly speaking, a care commodity. This care commodity aims at sustaining – and sometimes promoting – something called health. In the UK, many doctors, and especially 'junior' doctors, have been required to sell the care commodity they produce at a cheaper rate in worsened conditions of employment. At the same time, at some level, many will be aware of the ideological nature of the 'health' advice and support they are giving, and aware that this may be different from truly meaningful, health-giving advice and support. Without finding ways to resist, problems can deepen with doctors increasingly alienated from the care commodity they produce, from the patients they serve and ultimately from themselves. This is not a healthy situation to be in, neither for the doctors nor for the societies they serve. This is rooted in capitalist society such that permanent solutions can only derive from radical social change.

With this in mind, let us return to the concepts of dominant paradigms and paradigm shift developed by Kuhn in *The Structure of Scientific Revolutions*. In a science context, Kuhn develops an analysis of how transformative scientific ideas occur, not through the gradual process of experimentation and data accumulation, not as a result of working within what he calls dominant 'paradigms' of accepted scientific thought and methodologies, but outside of 'normal science', as a result of a revolutionary leap forward. He calls these 'paradigm shifts'. By paradigm Kuhn basically means the set of accepted ideas and practices which organise and constrain development within a particular field of study: 'A set of recurrent and quasi-standard illustrations of various theories in the conceptual, observational and instrumental applications ... revealed in its textbooks, lectures and laboratory exercises. By studying them and by practicing with them the members of the corresponding community learn their trade.'[32]

Though developed as a tool to analyse shifts in natural sciences, the ideas are useful in the social sciences too. For example, in educational studies a movement known as the cognitive revolution moved studies away from a behaviourist approach to the acceptance of cognition as central to studying human behaviour. In economics, the Keynesian revolution is viewed as a major paradigm shift in macroeconomics. It would seem logical, therefore to apply Kuhn's approach to an analysis of revolutionary medical advance, with its combination of scientific and socio-political modalities.

The English Revolution between the 1630s and 1680s had a major impact on subsequent medical science and practice, setting the paths along which medical science progressed up to the French Revolution. At a societal level, the basis of such later fields of medically related study as demography and epidemiology have their roots in the approaches put in place during the revolutionary years.[33] For example, pioneer demographer, John Graunt, studied burial records created following the execution of Charles I, to write his *Natural and Political Observations ... upon the Bills of Mortality* (1662).[34]

Thomas Sydenham (1624–89) – the English Hippocrates – and the ideas and practices he developed came to prominence as a direct result of the social and political upheaval of the English Revolution. Eventually a captain in Parliament's New Model Army, he began the war as a relatively obscure physician whose methods and opinions were at odds with the Royal College of Physicians' methods and beliefs. His support for Cromwell and Parliament gained him political preferences during the Commonwealth period after 1650. His book, *Observationes Medicae*, became a standard textbook of medicine into the nineteenth century and his work influenced the thinking of French revolutionaries a hundred years later.[35] For Sydenham medicine was a craft which would progress through observation of patients and monitoring therapies: 'I became convinced that the physician who earnestly studies with his own eyes and not through the medium of books the natural phenomena of the different diseases, must necessarily excel in the art of discovering what, in any given case are the true indications as to the remedial measures that should be employed.'[36]

He developed new treatments for diseases, including smallpox, and was renowned for his use of laudanum. He was the first to use quinine-containing cinchona bark for the treatment of malaria which, as Porter points out, is the first effective drug.[37] Most forms of ill health, he insisted, had a definite type, comparable to the types of animal and vegetable species. Having been excluded from influencing medical knowledge before the English Revolution, the revolution set him free to develop his medical approach. His work changed the pathways along which British – and subsequently European – medical knowledge developed. Sydenham's development of the concept of a person's 'constitution' is interpreted by Foucault as a 'complex of a set of natural events; qualities of soil, climate, seasons, rain, drought, centres of pestilence, famine',[38] a conceptualisation of health constitutions determined by social environments. Acute diseases, like fevers and inflammations, he regarded as useful and curative reactions by the body in defence against an 'injurious influence operating from without', an incredibly modern and insightful analysis. In this, he followed the Hippocratic teaching as well as the Hippocratic practice of watching and aiding natural crises.

The *Observationes Medicae* is a close study of the various fevers and other acute illnesses of London over a series of years, and their differences from year to year and from season to season, together with references to the prevailing weather. This body of observations were then used to map the epidemic constitution of the year or season. He attempted to develop longitudinal studies in order to analyse a totality of the combination of social and natural causes of disease at play. The type of the acute disease varied, he found, according to the year and season, and the right treatment could not be adopted until the type was known.[39] There had been nothing of this stature and insight in medical literature since Hippocrates. Sydenham's effort to tie treatment deductively to observable phenomena, and his concern for epidemic variations, were the forerunners to the careful, bedside observation of disease. He was the first modern doctor with a bedside manner. Sydenham's emphasis on the healing power of nature, and methodical treatment designed to work with that nature, created in his work a systematising and humanist tendency:

It is clearly impossible that a physician should discover those causes of disease that are not cognisable by the sense, so also it is unnecessary that he should attempt it. It is quite sufficient for him to know whence the mischief immediately arises … if he know rightly the cause by which it is immediately produced and if he can rightly discriminate between it and other diseases, he will be as certain to succeed in his attempts at a cure as if he had attended to idle and unprofitable searches in remote causes.[40]

Sydenham's work lifted the level on which medical science and practice progressed from then on. The dominant, feudal health paradigm, overseen by the Royal Society, shifted. The social and political upheavals of the English Revolution contextualised and supported this, providing a period of ideological and political flux in which new ideas could be considered and flourish, moving the basis on which medical thought and practice took place to a new level. His work also had wider repercussions, having a major impact on the philosophies developed in the following years by John Locke, a close personal friend.[41]

As with the English and French Revolutions, the Russian Revolution had an impact on healthcare and health science. Following the Russian Revolution a wave of struggle spread around Europe and beyond up until the mid-1920s, with revolutionary upheaval and mass strike activity in, among other regions, Germany, Italy, the UK, Hungary, Ireland, Mexico and Egypt. This half decade of open class warfare throughout Europe and beyond, with energised and organised working-class organisation threatening the continued dominance of old elites, is the essential political and ideological backdrop to British debates over the nature of health and welfare provision right through to the end of World War II. The Russian Revolution struck fear into the hearts of ruling elites around the world, and in Britain alerted many of them of the need for reform. As Harold Laski, future chairman of the Labour Party, reflected in 1927: 'The world has to find a response to the promise of communism in alternative forms, or it will discover that neither the crimes nor the follies of the Russian experiment will lessen the power to compel kindred action. In other words, the only way to avoid communism is to prove by public policy that it is unnecessary.'[42]

This idea of public policy as an alternative to communism is a theme to which I return below. In terms of developing approaches and systems to address the health needs of populations, by the 1930s the USSR led the way, which is amazing given the backward nature of pre-revolution Russian society. Writing in *Red Medicine: Socialised Health in Soviet Russia* in 1934, Sir Arthur Newsholme, formerly principle medical officer of the Local Government Board of England and Wales wrote of the:

Thousands of impressions of the means by which Russians in towns are helped to keep well and happy through a combination of abundant recreation and sports with a unique system of public health and medicine which in planning and to a large extent in accomplishment is more comprehensive and better unified than any we have found in making our surveys of other countries.[43]

Newsholme and Kingsbury's survey of health services in the USSR paints a vivid picture of the advances made in a very short space of time. In the Tartar Republic, 20 hospitals had been built between 1917 and 1932; women doctors and professors played major roles in the development and running of all aspects of the service, such as Dr Sholova, deputy commissar for health; a network of polyclinics – or health centres – was established; the service was integrated across disciplines so that public health combined with clinical health ensuring a preventative approach to health issues rather than a specifically curative one; health insurance was paid through an industry levy, so that industries were responsible for paying for healthcare, not individuals; and all major factories had their own healthcare provision. Trainee doctors were chosen 'by committees of their fellow workers ... The choice depends greatly on the social occupation of the student, manual workers having a preference'.[44] Compare this to the situation in Britain where still, in the twenty-first century, less than 20 per cent of doctors enter the profession via a working-class education. Over 80 per cent of medical students come from households containing professionals or those in higher managerial roles, and more than a quarter from private schools.[45]

Russian health gains came at a social and political cost for the Russian population generally. By the 1920s Russia had become a state capitalist enterprise, entangled in a world of capitalism so that Russian workers' healthcare gains may well have been secured at the cost of political freedom of expression and more widespread persecution and repression. The Russian state developed the health provision observed by Newsholme and others not least to ensure a fit – and potentially pliant – workforce, the better to engage in the imperialist 'world tournament of nations', as Nikolai Bukharin puts it.[46] But this is not the central issue. The key point here is that Russia provided an alternative (planned) model to the 'rudderless drifting' of health provision in Britain and elsewhere. A final point on the Russian system: progress was all the more remarkable given the counter-revolutionary war of Western-backed armies in the years following 1917. Following that war famine ravaged the USSR, with an estimated six million people dying.[47] In these circumstances it became essential to develop health measures to address widespread outbreaks of cholera, dysentery, typhus and smallpox if the USSR was to survive at all. In these conditions, as reflected on by N.A. Semashko, commissar of health in 1923, the USSR was able to actually reduce child mortality rates, and quickly develop public health measures – like travelling dispensaries and a network of sanatoriums – to begin to bring disease under control. Semashko was very clear that:

All comrades must realise that it is in raising the public health, lies the best basis for a sound rebuilding of Russian economic life. The rebuilding of Russia cannot be carried through by a sick nation, by broad masses whose hygiene, physique and sanitary requirements are not well developed. In the great and heavy work of rebuilding Russia, the health standard of the Russian masses is of the very first importance.[48]

In the post-revolutionary USSR context the authorities were clear: the health of the individual was the responsibility of the state and on it the wealth and well-being of the USSR collective was dependent. The revolutionary break with the feudal order, and the needs of emergent Russian capitalism, contextualised the qualitative shift in medial practice. This modern, centralised and highly successful practice set the new global standards for centrally planned and resourced, community delivered healthcare – preventative as well as curative.

We might think of the example of 'health' discussed above and how doctors learn their trade through being active participants, albeit at times unknowingly, in the propagation of an idea of health which is deeply ideological. During social revolutions, old ideologies, ideas and even the language to describe them become strained. The very foundational basis on which the terms and ideas of healthcare practice –as shown earlier in the examples of the English, French and Russian revolutions – no longer make sense in a new social context and they are junked, to be replaced by new potentials.

During each revolutionary period the movement in thought, systems and scientific and social practice was, as Kuhn argues, away from previous conceptions of the world dictated by the 'normal science' of medical practice. In England in the 1630s and 1640s the continued forward march to power of the nascent English bourgeoisie became threatened by the rearguard defence of royal privilege by Charles I and his allies, throwing British society as a whole into crisis; France at the end of the eighteenth century was the centre of European autocratic monarchy which frustrated the aspirations of the French bourgeoisie at a time of economic crisis caused by the outmoded and economically inefficient nature of the old, feudal order, setting in train a period of social crisis resulting in the victory of a modern bourgeois class; in Russia, the slaughter of World War I served to illustrate the economic and political backwardness of the autocratic monarchy there, which was unable to answer the basic subsistence and survival needs of the Russian population, resulting in a workers' revolution led by Lenin and the Bolsheviks, offering – but ultimately unable to deliver – a new form of socialist society in radical response.

In each of these revolutions the intervention of the masses was central. Whether that be the workers and peasants gathered together in the Red Army and soviets during the Russian Revolution, the shock troops of the Sans-culottes in the street battles and at the National Assembly in France or the 'Middling Sort' of the English Civil War, small independent famers, yeomen and artisans, tradesmen, husbandmen and labourers, released from feudal ideological bondage and taking the lead in the ranks of the New Model Army as Agitators, and at an ideological level reinterpreting the words of the Bible to support their cause. As an unnamed professional preacher of pre-revolutionary days exclaimed: 'But whence come they now, from the schooles of the Prophets? No, many, of them from mechanike trades as one from a stable from currying his horses; another from a stall from cobbling his shoes ... These take upon them to reveal their secrets of almighty God, to open and shut heaven, to save soules.'[49]

Through this expanded dialogue ideas at all levels change. For Kuhn, revolutions in science 'change the domain, change even the very language in which we speak',[50] and this is recognised by Foucault in his analysis of medical discourse and change during the French Revolution, though he does not attribute this change to the revolutionary process itself.[51] The change even of language is explicitly recognised as a feature of the English Revolution when Petegorsky writes, referencing the great English Revolution historian R.H. Tawney, 'Ethical and religious ideals no longer corresponded to the social reality they were intended to regulate'; in the words of Tawney, 'their practical ineffectiveness paved the way for their theoretical abandonment'.[52]

In each of the cases cited above a 'paradigm shift' occurred, moving medical science and practice onto a new plain. Only the force of the social and political upheaval could, in each case, loosen the grip of an old order constraining innovation and development, and start to provide solutions to the changing health needs of whole populations in a new age.

8

Legislating for Better Health?

History shows that social revolutions fundamentally shift science and health paradigms, moving the potential for improving health onto a different plain. But away from such cataclysmic events, how has health improvement occurred? Various arguments have been made over time to explain health improvements: from those crediting medical advance, to those focusing on general economic growth and its impact on health, to more modern ideas which consider the impact of modern social policy.

Up until the twenty-first century, demographic transition theory (DTM) has provided a conceptual framework for understanding health improvement at population levels. DTM uses historical population trends of birth and death rates to argue that population growth rates cycle through stages based on economic growth. Each stage is characterised by a specific relationship between birth rate (number of annual births per 1,000 people) and death rate (number of annual deaths per 1,000 people). As these rates change in relation to each other, their impact affects a country's total population. The model claims that global populations move through distinct stages, from stage 1 where death and birth rates are both high, producing relative equilibrium such as in pre-industrial populations; to stage 5 where there are more older people than young, producing the kind of ageing population scenarios critiqued in Chapter 6. Central to DTM is the idea that economic growth is the driver of rising populations. DTM has been criticised on the basis of its many methodological problems, as well as on the basis of its historical inaccuracy. Today, it is generally regarded as, at best, a set of generalisations rather than a unified theory.[1]

From the 1950s, another version of population expansion through health improvement based on economic growth came to prominence, the so-called McKeown thesis. In 1955 Thomas McKeown and Robert Brown analysed the relation of medicine and medical advance to the increase in Britain's population from the late eighteenth century. Starting with the fact that population growth had occurred in the majority of more economically advanced countries, with different timing and rates of increase, McKeown and Brown began by questioning the role of the medical profession in health improvements. Up to this point it had been largely accepted that improvements in medical science had been a key driver of health improvement across populations, a theory which helped to justify focusing financial and other health-related resources on the major teaching hospitals, to the detriment of medical research and, McKeown and Brown argued, of a more preventative public health service.

McKeown and Brown pointed to the fact that doctors had virtually no effective drugs at their disposal during the key periods of population growth, that medical skills were limited and that pre-Listerian surgery was barbaric and often led to death from sepsis or shock.[2] In the UK during this period, hospitals were places to which people went only as a last resort. Roy Porter's monumental study of medicine illustrates the piecemeal nature of advance in UK medicine during this period, influenced by but lagging far behind medical advance in post-revolutionary France. Porter recounts the experiences of a young trainee doctor: 'I entered St Bart-holomew's Hospital … there was very little, or no, personal guidance; the demonstrators had some private pupils, who they "ground" for the College examinations, but these were only a small portion of the school; the surgeons had apprentices, to whom they seldom taught more than other students; for the most part, the students guided themselves.'[3]

Patients often died due to hospital-acquired infections and the general lack of skill and knowledge of doctors. For McKeown and Brown this ruled out the idea that medical practice could have had anything like the supposed impact on public health and population growth. McKeown felt smallpox vaccination was the exception that proved the rule, representing the isolated high point of medical intervention in the early period. It could not alone account for the nineteenth-century population rise.[4] The McKeown thesis overturned the idea that medical advance had been principally responsible for declines in mortality, and McKeown conclusively proves that medical science could not have accounted for more than a tiny fraction of any improvement in mortality that occurred before the 1930s, when sulphonamides and antibacterial agents finally arrived.[5]

In place of the medical explanations of mortality decline, McKeown proposed what Szreter has called a 'nutritional determinism'.[6] McKeown's analysis of the epidemiological evidence suggested to him that the major factor was a 'rising standard of living, of which the most significant feature was improved diet'.[7] For McKeown, rising populations were due more to decreases in mortality rates than to increases in fertility, and this was primarily due to better diets.[8] This, in turn, resulted from economic growth. McKeown felt economic growth in and of itself contextualised and crucially determined population growth.

In order to develop his thesis, McKeown grouped individual diseases into four broad etiological categories, according to what modern medical science understands to be the main pathways of transmission involved in the spread of disease. These are airborne micro-organisms; water- and food-borne micro-organisms and other micro-organisms; other conditions. As Szreter shows, with this system of classification McKeown argued that any improvement in general health expressed in rising populations must be due to one of the following:

(1) An autonomous decline in the virulence of the micro-organism itself.

(2) An improvement in the overall environment so as to reduce the chances of initial exposure to potentially harmful organisms, either from (a) scientific advances in immunization techniques or (b) public health policies designed to sanitise the urban environment – something he termed 'municipal sanitation' or 'hygiene improvements'.

(3) Improvements in the human victim's defensive resources after initial exposure to hostile organisms either as a result of (a) the development of effective scientific methods of treating symptoms or (b) via an increase in the level and quality of the exposed population's average nutritional intake – that is, better and more abundant food, thereby improving the individual's own natural defences.[9]

On the balance of his analysis of the evidence, and building on a growing consensus that medical advance was not responsible, McKeown concluded that more and better quality food was responsible for improvements in mortality rates, and his thesis has largely been accepted by academics and policymakers since the late 1970s.

More recently, during the first decades of the twenty-first century, due in large part to the work of the Cambridge Group, an alternative analysis has developed. This attributes population growth during the nineteenth century not primarily to improved food intake, not even to improved mortality rates, but rather to increased fertility rates resulting in large part from improvements in sanitation. This line of arguments points to policy-driven changes which made crowded urban environments healthier to live in and supportive of better health for mothers and infants. In short, the Cambridge Group's thesis is that action at local government level during the mid to late nineteenth century to address the sewage disposal and general sanitation requirements of the overcrowded cities that had grown during the first half of the nineteenth century improved the life expectancies of, in particular, the industrial working class.[10] Coupled with a now-accepted longer-term trend for people to marry and have children earlier – thus increasing birth rates – this political intervention into the social conditions, or social determinants, of health was responsible for the better health of populations and subsequently its growth. Szreter shows that as a result of improved sanitation, waterborne diseases decreased, with the last great cholera outbreak occurring in the mid-1850s. McKeown disputes the centrality of this by pointing to the fall in incidence of airborne diseases, such as smallpox and scarlet fever, over this period, which McKeown attributes to the strengthening of the body's immune systems resulting from improved diet consequent upon generally rising living standards through economic growth. His criticism is that improvements in sanitation cannot account for the drop in these. In response, Szreter shows that the composite of airborne diseases, including bronchitis, pneumonia and influenza (the second most important cause of death during the mid-1800s) actually increased during the latter part of this period, from accounting for over 10 per cent of all deaths up to 20 per cent by 1901. This undermines McKeown's thesis that improved diets strengthened immune systems.

Beyond generalised references to 'standard of living' improvements, McKeown plays down the impact of improvements in the social determinants of health resulting from socio-political developments. Improvements in working conditions, housing, education and others did not arise as a 'natural' consequence of economic expansion as McKeown wants. They resulted from specific phases of demands and action by working people, at times enacted into local and national legislation by their representatives in local government. McKeown's thesis, as Szreter conclusively shows, fails to acknowledge this question of agency.

Numerous government and independent reports during the period show that overcrowded conditions of living, sleeping and working increased as industrialisation and urbanisation intensified.[11] This was reversed not through generalised rising wage levels and improved 'standards of living' but by resistance and pressure for improvements from working people passing into law via Factory and Workshop Acts, Housing and Crowding Acts and the enforcement of building regulations and by-laws.

While McKeown's exploration of the historical record was effective in showing as false the claims regarding population growth through medical advance (the orthodoxy of his day), in focusing on this McKeown downplayed the role of human agency. What his thesis leaves us with is the idea that health improves as a result of the 'invisible hand' of rising living standards, conceived as an impersonal and inevitable by-product of general economic growth. McKeown's thesis prepares the way for what became known in the 1980s as the 'trickle down' approach, with health improving as an inevitable consequence of elements of a society enriching themselves, and something Szreter's work conclusively refutes.

In place of this, the Cambridge Group analysis recognises the role of human agency in health improvement. Their focus is on the impact of improvements in sanitation and, more specifically, the role of local authorities in pioneering this. Their analysis details the activities of central and local government in acting to make cities safer and healthier through public interventions in sewage and sanitation systems, and through acting to improve living and working conditions generally. As Szreter argues, 'the period from the late 1830s to 1875 came to be seen as encompassing a "heroic age" of pioneering advances in public health activism and legislation'.[12] Public figures like William Farr, and doctors Neil Arnott, James Kay and Thomas Southwood Smith, accompanied Edwin Chadwick's 'Sanitary Idea' realised through the first Public Health Act of 1848. This central government lead influenced later initiatives at local level, when, as Anthony Whol makes clear, it was during the last 30 years of the century that the most significant improvements and concrete applications of preventative health measures occurred.[13]

In the 1860s governments began to record and set targets for local districts, with comparisons in terms of numbers of lives needlessly lost in the 'Black Spots' relative to the 'Healthy Districts' around the UK. As Szreter points out, 'Commerce and business was believed to be attracted to those cities with the lowest death-rates'.[14] Local authorities began to recognise that not only did their newly enlarged electorate want and need improvements in living conditions, they were likely to attract capital by doing so. Both the working class and the employing class wanted welfare-based change. As I showed in Chapter 7, the second half of the nineteenth century saw a shift in attitudes and policy across Europe as countries moved away from the 'Manchester model' towards one focused on developing a more stable and healthy workforce. Developments outlined above can be seen in this light. Centrally, not only was key legislation passed but at a more fundamental level the idea was put into practice that governments at central and local level were required to consider the collective needs of the population in general, not just the needs of the employing class as had been the case. But this realisation by UK and European governments did not result from their general feelings of goodwill to all men. It was contextualised by nearly half a century of open and often violent class struggle.

Joseph Chamberlain was a key political figure of this period, illustrative of general trends and shifts in class dynamics over the mid-to-late nineteenth century. Mayor of Birmingham between 1873 and 1876, he started life as a radical Liberal and ended as a Conservative. He was associated with a number of acts of parliament shaping a more interventionist and welfare-driven approach towards the health of working people. As Birmingham mayor he first developed the ideas of 'gas and water municipal socialism', ideas later taken on and developed by the Fabians Sydney and Beatrice Webb. He argued that failure to spend on the town's environment was a false economy, undermining the health of the working people on which the town's wealth depended – although, of course, being a long-time and staunch member of Birmingham's employing class, he didn't quite put it like that! Regardless, the key point here is that the Cambridge Group's analysis, with the focus on political actors, situates the improvements in health that resulted in population growth unequivocally in what people do. For the Cambridge Group, the key element in terms of health improvements over the period was the legislation passed, in particular from the mid-1840s onwards. It is important, therefore, to be clear about what underpins and drives this kind of social policy.

A critical social policy approach[15] understands social policy in general and welfare policy in particular as resulting from the conflict between labour and capital. Accordingly, policy results from: 'The struggle of the working class against their exploitation; the requirements of industrial capitalism ... for a more efficient environment in which to operate; recognition by the property owners of the price that has to be paid for political security'.[16] This produces social policy with a dual nature, both potentially addressing social inequality and acting as a means of social control according to the 'requirements of the capitalist economy'.[17] Historically shifting patterns of, for example, welfare provision can be understood in these terms,[18] with a capitalist class supporting the need for welfare investment when it suits their interests and opposing them when it does not:

> From the late nineteenth century to around 1920, as foreign competition and labour unrest intensified, many influential employers began to argue for state welfare as a means of social control and as a contribution to economic efficiency ... When mass unemployment took the edge off labour militancy and guaranteed a supply of labour, employers became more sensitive to the costs of welfare.[19]

Pioneers of critical social policy Peter Taylor-Goody and Mary Dale identify three ways in which class interests are expressed in welfare policy. First, working-class pressure leads to concessions from the government, especially in liberal democracies; second, the government formulates and prosecutes the long-term interests of capital, either by initiating policies, or by adapting the concessions it has granted under the pressure of class struggle to the needs of capital; third, the working class and the capitalist class may both see certain reforms as being in their interests. This gives us a framework with which to understand health improvements in the UK in the second half of the nineteenth century.

In the UK between 1830 and 1848 were 18 years of social upheaval, a period through which Chartism – the first mass workers' movement in history – developed. In three waves and culminating in 1848, Chartism helped to set the context in which social policy in the following years developed. In 1848 revolutionary struggle defined not only the UK but the whole of Europe, with uprisings in France, Italy, Germany and the countries of the old Habsburg monarchy including Austria, Hungary, Bohemia and Slovakia. As well as this Switzerland, Denmark, Romania, Poland and Ireland experienced social and political upheaval. Typically, across Europe these movements were collusions between classes, with the rising bourgeois class taking the lead. The Chartist movement was different. The movements formalised numerous specifically working-class demands ranging from a call for the UK to move to a paper money system from the Birmingham Union, to the dissolution of the Poor Laws made by the Great Northern Union, led by the most radical of the Chartist leaders Fergus O'Connor. All of the versions of the Charter, from which the movement took its name, argued for the extension of the franchise to include working-class men.

Historians have argued and continue to argue over the causes and consequences of this period of upheaval mid-way through the nineteenth century and here is definitely not the place to attempt to analyse that. What is relevant, however, is to try to understand how this period of open class warfare across Europe (especially, for our purposes, in the UK) influenced the health of UK populations over the years following it. The widespread nature and intensity of the class struggle of the period between 1830 and 1848 in the UK has been well documented over time,[20] with the highpoints of support for Chartism probably coming in 1839, 1842 and culminating in 1848 when anywhere between 15,000 and 300,000 – depending on whether you believe the estimates of the police or those of the demonstration organisers – gathered at Kennington Common in south London in support of the Chartist Convention. Millions of working people – the organisers claimed six million people for the Charter of 1848 – signed petitions in support of universal manhood suffrage, nearly a quarter of the entire UK population at that time. The 1839 phase of the movement saw mass rioting take place in Newport, south Wales and in Birmingham, with the Bull Ring Riots of July that year, both forcibly repressed.

For our purposes, trying to understand how the class struggle of this period contextualised the health of populations and future social policy influencing that health, it is important to understand how different classes behaved. For the revolutionary upheavals across Europe historians and commentators have concluded that an emergent bourgeois class, variously described as a 'middle' or 'liberal' class, withdrew from pressing the full extent of their claims on social and political power. Historian Peter Stearns, for example, argues that 'the social class that had provided leadership to all the major revolutions withdrew from the arena. The intellectual mood capable of generating the spirit that could convert ideology to revolutionary action was gone ... Advancing industrialisation in fact made change inevitable. But revolution was no longer the vehicle for change'.[21] Writing at the time Karl Marx, specifically discussing events in France, vividly exemplifies how post-revolutionary states were able to co-opt the old social and political structures and social actors into the new: 'The seignorial privileges of the landowners and towns became transformed into so many attributes of state power, the feudal dignitaries into paid officials, and the motley pattern of conflicting medieval plenary powers into the regulated plan of a state authority whose work is divided and centralised as in a factory'.[22] The European uprisings ended in compromise states, and for Marx and many others this marked the end of the bourgeoisie as a revolutionary class.

The Chartist movement differed from this pattern in that its leadership was either drawn from or depended for their support upon the working class. In his study of the Birmingham Union, Flick points to the fact that, by 1838 at least, 'the middle classes ... were unwilling to unite with the workers in demand for further constitutional change'.[23] The Birmingham Union was the most moderate of the three great centres of Chartism at this time, the others being the London Working Men's Association, which largely took a similarly moderate stance, and the Great Northern Union under O'Connor's revolutionary leadership. When it came to support for the cause of the working man from the middle classes, what was true of Birmingham was doubly true of the other regions: 'When a few, scattered political unions did appear in the country, they were mostly radical ones of the working-classes with little or no middle-class membership'.[24] As Marxist historian John Saville argues, it was in 1848 'that it was demonstrated beyond question and doubt, the complete and solid support of the middling strata to the defence of existing institutions' and against the radicalisation of the working class.[25]

Though Birmingham and London were what became known as 'moral force' regions – determined to press their case on the basis of the justifiable and moral nature of their appeals – because of the revolutionary nature of the Great Northern Union, once in alliance all three regions carried with them the implicit threat of armed uprising. For example, on a speaking tour of the north, the leadership of the Birmingham Union found that the Great Northern Union had 5,000 guns stashed away in potential support of a revolution which many thought would be justified to repeal the Poor Law.[26] In 1848 in the months after the Kennington Common demonstration, historical evidence shows that Chartists were armed and drilling in the West Riding and formulating political plots in support of insurrection in London.[27] For the first time in the history of industrial capitalism in the UK an independent working-class movement, organised on a national basis with articulate and effective leaders and carrying with them the threat of armed insurrectionary violence, appeared to press their demands on the employing class and the state.

Thus, we arrive at the classic context, described by critical social policy, for the development of policy and legislation, with a working-class struggling against its exploitation, industrial capitalism seeking the 'most efficient environment' to operate in and an employing class which recognises concessions need to be made to secure its political position. In the economically expanding context of the years following Chartism what this in effect meant was an explosion in trade union membership from a little over 100,000 in 1850 to well over a million members by 1874. This period also saw the rise of the so-called 'new unionism', with older, more traditional unions often amalgamating to form larger, national organisations. These new unions, like the Amalgamated Society of Engineers, the model on which many new unions were based, employed full-time union officials to organise workers and increasingly take on bargaining roles with the employing class, establishing themselves as a layer of arbiters between classes.[28]

At the level of health-related policy and legislation this was a golden age both in terms of specific public health legislation (as discussed earlier), but also with regard to child employment and health and safety at work legislation. Following Chartism there were Factory Acts in 1844, 1847, 1850, 1853, 1860, 1864, two in 1867 and 1878. As Marx said at the time, in particular referencing the Factory Act of 1847 which put a limit of ten hours on the daily labour of women and children in textile mills: 'It was the first time that in broad daylight the political economy of the middle class succumbed to the political economy of the working-class'.[29]

This legislation massively improved working conditions and general levels of health and health outcomes, and increased the expectations of the working class in the UK and beyond, breaking the grip of the outmoded Manchester model and setting the standards for working conditions in Germany and other European countries. It set into law strict limits on the employment of child labour, setting the way for the Education Acts that followed, both of which, by removing children from the health-threatening intensity of workplaces, improved child survival rates and health generally. Before Chartism the appalling living conditions in urban areas had been well documented, but it took until after Chartism for Chadwick's 'sanitary idea' to be implemented in 1848, as local politicians began to understand the necessity of addressing the needs and demands of the (now expanded) electorate they served, as well as the longer-term needs of the employing class for a sustainable and able-to-work workforce. It is in this general context that we can understand the events in Birmingham to which Szreter refers when he discusses the contribution to public health of Joseph Chamberlain.

The municipal socialism of the mid-1870s, pioneered by Chamberlain, was an outgrowth and an expression at local level of this need for social policy to fuse the needs of working people with those of the employing class. Chamberlain experienced at first hand the strength of the Birmingham proletariat. In August 1866 he took part in a 250,000-strong demonstration through Birmingham in support of an extension of the franchise, ending in a public meeting. He recalled that 'men poured into the hall, black as they were from the factories ... the people were packed together like herrings'[30] to listen to speeches in support of the vote. A year later the minority Conservative government passed the 1867 Reform Act, doubling the electorate to nearly 2.5 million. His 'gas and water municipal socialism' idea was, as Szreter shows, a major step forward in terms of public health in the city. As we have seen, this benefited both working-class people in improvements made to their living conditions, as well as the employing class in ensuring a more stable and reliable workforce fit for exploitation more efficiently over a longer period of time, as Labisch shows.

Chamberlain was one among many of the employing class at the time to realise that the maintenance of a relatively healthy and fit-to-work working class was the essential condition of a productive labour force. As a result, from the mid-1840s onwards there is a long history of employers accepting as necessary the concessions made as a result of working-class pressure. In the cases where employers actually have to make real concessions, there is an acknowledgement expressed through history that this is part of what Chamberlain himself described in 1885 as the ransom to be paid for avoiding more serious attacks on the employing class's general privileges.[31]

The term 'municipal socialism' is in itself intriguing. By this time, the 1870s, several versions of socialist ideas were taking shape and influencing political life. That Chamberlain – certainly no socialist – should choose this phrase illustrates another political and ideological tendency of this post-revolutionary period, that of the weaker version of the dominant ideology thesis. An idea developed by Tom Bottomore,[32] this concept details 'the capacity of a dominant ideology to inhibit and confuse the development of the counter-ideology of a subordinate class'. As a range of socialist ideas took shape, the concept of municipal socialism, used here by Chamberlain and taken on by the Fabians, was to suggest the possibility that socialist aims could be achieved by working through already existing state and local government structures. The idea suggests there is no need for independent working-class organisation, simply a need to vote in able representatives. As Canguilhem puts it in another context, we might understand the health legislation of the latter part of the nineteenth century as: 'The expression of the relative efficiency of a regime invented to channel and smother social antagonisms, of a political machine acquired by modern societies in order to delay, without finally being able to prevent, the transformation of inconsistencies into crisis.'[33]

9

Who's WHO?

In Chapter 4 I explained the role played by WHO in developing the social determinants of health approach to a higher level. Here I explore whether the approach taken by WHO in pursuit of developing this concept through policy and international collaboration is a useful one. In brief, it asks can WHO solve global health inequality?

During the course of the twenty-first century, WHO has been central to developing the ideas of the social determinants of health which, I have argued, is a useful analytical tool for understanding health outcomes in history, and potentially for developing strategies to address health inequalities and the 'health deficit'. In 2003 WHO constructed a list of the major determinants, which was later built on by Canadian academics, where public health issues have consistently occupied positions of importance in both academic study and government policy.[1] In 2008 WHO CSDH published a report entitled *Closing the Gap in a Generation*, setting out an agenda and draft strategies to improve global health. In this, child labour and child health is a particular concern to WHO's agenda. Investment in early child development (ECD) is described in the report as 'one of the most powerful that countries can make in terms of reducing the escalating chronic disease burden in adults'.[2] The report highlights the continuing high death rates among children from disadvantaged backgrounds worldwide, mostly in LMICs but also including HICs like the UK. The report points to the ten million preventable infant deaths occurring every year as a result of poor social conditions.[3] As a means of addressing this, *Closing the Gap* suggests more rigorous and consistent strategies for ECD.

An example of ECD with which readers might be familiar are the UK Labour governments' Sure Start programmes of 1997–2010. These were targeted in localities of higher than average need and provided a range of support and advice for families with children under the age of four, and often highly valued by the service users. To what extent Sure

Start benefited as a source of professional advice and to what extent it provided a convenient and affordable space for mothers to pass on advice and share experiences between parents, as they always have throughout history, is a moot point. Initially, the programmes were government funded and directed, but after 2004 local authority-run programmes largely became Sure Start Centres which increasingly morphed into individualised registered charities as part of the broader independent voluntary sector. With the 'tapering' of the original government funding, numerous centres closed such that the original architect of the scheme, Norman Glass, became very critical of the lack of resourcing and the diminution of democratic control.[4] This gradual reduction in local government funding and the offloading of services to the voluntary sector was part of a broader and longer-established agenda of 'outsourcing' of previously run local authority services. Outlining its intent to focus attention on addressing health inequalities from the early years onwards, via ECD strategies, *Closing the Gap* states: 'Social inequalities in early life contribute to inequities in health later on ... Children from disadvantaged backgrounds are more likely to do poorly in school and subsequently, as adults, are more likely to have lower incomes and higher fertility rates.'[5]

These findings, and of particular interest the correlation between low incomes and high fertility rates, are based largely on the findings of one piece of research by Grantham-McGregor, a weakness WHO readily concedes.[6] The argument, though, is at least superficially seductive. Surely, if WHO could play a role in ensuring a better education for poor children, wouldn't this give them a better chance at a higher-paid job, lifting them out of poverty through dint of their own skills and efforts fitting them for better employment? To this end WHO suggest setting up 'inter-agency mechanisms' to coordinate ECD to safeguard and promote opportunities and ensure lower fertility rates. Currently, the range of agencies already involved in intervening in the ECD of LMIC children includes the UNDP, Office of the UN High Commissioner for Refugees, UNICEF, UN Population Fund, World Food Programme, UN Human Settlements Programme, International Labour Organization, the Food and Agriculture Organisation of the UN, UN Educational, Scientific and Cultural Organisation, WHO itself, Joint UN Programme on HIV/AIDS, the World Bank, International Monetary Fund and International Organisation for Migration, along with a range of civil society – by which the document means independent or voluntary sector organisations – and other 'partners'. This is an impressive body of stakeholders, though there doesn't seem to have been room for what might be called 'service users'. The cynical might suggest that perhaps the sum total of salaries being generated by this array of agencies might go some way to addressing some of the problems they want to debate.

That aside, an example of one of these inter-agency mechanisms in action, so to speak, might be the Standing Committee on Nutrition (SCN). Set up as a result of this WHO initiative the SCN has been in operation for over a decade now. During that time, as WHO reported in 2017, 'Obesity has reached epidemic proportions globally, with at least 2.8 million people dying each year as a result of being overweight or obese. Once associated with high-income countries, obesity is now also prevalent in low- and middle-income countries.'[7] Clearly, there are forces beyond the reach of WHO committees, which are having a greater impact than the SCN could ever hope to despite its very impressive backing from so many international agencies.

If it is failing on diet, what about WHO's links between better education and better employment? It is not inevitable that a better education automatically leads to better paid and secure employment. For example, research in 2018 shows that university graduates in the US, UK and elsewhere are no longer guaranteed access to better employment simply as a result of higher educational qualifications.[8] What of the supporting assertion made in *Closing the Gap* that lower educational attainment leads to higher fertility rates? There is a long and uncomfortable history of the question of what has been described as the 'problem' of higher fertility rates of people living in poverty which has its roots very firmly in the eugenics movement of the late nineteenth and early twentieth centuries. Here is not the place to explore the infamous history of the eugenics movement, but suffice to say central to its aims and strategies over the 60 or 70 years of influence across Europe and North America was the control of the fertility rates of poor people. Writing on behalf of the UK's social hygiene movement in 1938, eugenicist Richard Titmuss, discussing what he termed 'the Social Problem Group', explained that from this group 'all too many of our criminals, paupers, degenerates, unemployables and defectives are recruited'.[9] John Maynard Keyes, whose economic ideas set the basis for governments and social policy globally following World War II, remained an avid eugenicist throughout his life.

Ideas and assumptions drawn from the eugenics movement underscored the post-World War II American Population Control Movement through to the 1970s, having a major impact on global aid policy throughout the period.[10]

Employment is at the heart of the relationship between poverty and fertility rates. Drawing on the work of Marmot and Wilkinson,[11] *Closing the Gap* says that 'good' employment can have beneficial effects on health. In order to attempt to influence this, the WHO document calls for a 'Healthy Living Wage', stating: 'Providing a living wage that takes into account the real and current cost of living for health requires supportive economic and social policy that is regularly updated and is based on the costs of health needs including adequate nutritious food, shelter, water and sanitation, and social participation.'[12] The advice, however, comes with a further consideration: 'In low-income countries, competitive advantage is heavily dependent on low labour costs, and this may be compromised if provision of a regularly updated decent living wage becomes a statutory requirement.'[13] It would seem the only way to read this is that WHO recommends that a healthy living wage should be a statutory requirement unless a particular country would lose 'competitive advantage' by doing so. In other words, in order to remain 'competitive' countries should be supported in paying below a healthy living wage to their workers. This is clearly contradictory.

Let us look at the Malthusian muddle with regard to 'low incomes and high fertility rates' which seemingly continues to inform WHO perspectives. Malthusian ideas have been debated since the beginning of the industrial revolution. Very briefly, Thomas Malthus was a British commentator at the turn of the nineteenth century, who stated over the course of his three key documents that the problem at the heart of continued growth of the UK economy was the question of overpopulation. For Malthus and his supporters too many poor people were chasing too few resources and were subsequently a social burden and block on prosperity. On the basis of less than rigorous research he argued that populations grew in geometric progression while food production grew in arithmetic progression. A geometric progression is a sequence of numbers where each number after the first results from multiplying the previous one by a fixed number. For example, in the sequence 2, 10, 50, 250, 1250, the common ratio is 5. An arithmetic progression is a sequence of numbers where the difference between them is constant. For example, in the sequence 2, 5, 8, 11, 14, 17, the common difference is 3. We can see from this that, using the Malthus method, populations will grow faster than the supply of food leading to food shortages and starvation. He theorised that this 'correction' occurs in the form of positive and preventative checks. These checks would lead to the Malthusian catastrophe, which would bring the population back to a 'sustainable level'.[14]

Population growth would depress wages, causing mortality to rise due to famine, war or disease – in short, 'misery'. Malthus called this the 'positive' check. Depressed wages were also likely to cause prostitution and other 'vices'; this he called the 'preventive' check. Since population potentially grew more rapidly than the economy, it was always held in check by 'misery and vice', which were therefore the inevitable human lot. Economic progress could help only temporarily since population could soon grow to its new equilibrium level, where misery and vice would again hold it in check. Only through moral restraint did Malthus believe that humanity might avoid this fate, and he thought this an unlikely outcome.[15]

Writing at the same time as Malthus, Marx and Engels were angrily critical of his work, attacking it as plagiarised and deeply ideological: 'Malthus' book on Population was a tract against the French Revolution ... It was an apology for the poverty of the working-classes. The theory was a plagiarism of Townsend ... His Principals of Political Economy was a tract in the interests of capitalists against workers ... a plagiarism of Adam Smith.[16] Against the Malthusian idea that populations somehow develop in isolation from the economic and material environments they find themselves in, Marx and Engels argue that populations develop in response to this environment. They refer to the father of capitalist economics, Adam Smith, in so doing pointing to Smith's argument that 'the demand for men, like that for any other commodity, necessarily regulates the production of men, quickens it when it goes on too slowly, and stops it when it advances too fast'.[17] Through this critique Marx and Engels develop the idea of a 'surplus population' or a 'reserve army of labour'. Engels' description of this surplus population also serves as an illustration of the process of exploitation at the heart of its creation:

> Surplus population is engendered rather by the competition of the workers among themselves, which forces each separate worker to labour as much each day as his strength can possibly admit. If a man-

ufacturer can employ ten hands nine hours daily he can employ nine if each works ten hours, and the tenth goes hungry. And if a manufacturer can force the nine hands to work an extra hour daily for the same wages by threatening to discharge them at a time when the demand for hands is not very great, he discharges the tenth and saves so much wages.[18]

High fertility rates are contextualised by the specific wealth development needs of a specific country or region. As Engels makes clear, the employing class benefits from having a supply of labour in excess to his or her immediate needs, using this reserve army of labour to hold down average wages and gain, as the WHO document succinctly puts it, 'competitive advantage'. As I argue above, globally child labour is endemic. Children go to find work because their families need every ounce of additional income in order for any semblance of a family to survive, as they always have in a class society. In the name of protecting 'competitive advantage', WHO and the plethora of other international agencies connected with them perpetuate this poverty and the 'high fertility rates' it targets. It is the market-driven demand for cheap labour that governs fertility rates, not high fertility rates developing in isolation that hold people in poverty as Malthus – and WHO – would have us believe.

Market-driven requirements almost completely beyond the control of international bodies like WHO impact on LMICs in a number of other ways too, and I finish by briefly looking at two – the choices of what is produced in specific countries and regions and the influence over this and other decisions by multinational companies and so-called 'civil society' agencies.

In Chapter 4 I discussed child labour in sugar cane growing globally. Sugar cane is a cash crop, grown not for an indigenous population to eat but for a government – or other private company – to sell. Cash crops have been critiqued for an extensive range of reasons, including the growing of such crops being an expression of colonialism, replacing traditional, pre-colonialist agricultural practice that guaranteed societal and family food security. It has also been criticised on the basis of the negative consequences for indigenous populations because of its association with large-scale, capital-intensive industries on potentially high-yield land.[19] The general gist of these arguments is that cash crops grown for profit have replaced useful food grown for local populations to eat for reasons of commerce and economics, at the cost of poverty and the increased exploitation of indigenous populations, as well as the declining standards of health coterminous with these developments.

The global consequences of the adoption of modern food methods and technologies on indigenous populations and foodstuff production have been severe. In India over the course of the twenty-first century hunger, poverty and suicide rates have all grown as modern food production techniques linked to global food markets produce an 'over-production' crisis. As agroecologists Eric Holt-Gimenez and Raj Patel show: 'In 2001, with granaries so full of surplus that Indian authorities proposed dumping them into the sea, hunger deaths were reported in 12 Indian states – deaths unheard of since the 1960s.'[20] Africa between 1970 and the twenty-first century has moved from being a net exporter of food to a net importer, with, in 2009, almost every country on the continent having to import up to 25 per cent of its food.[21]

Cash crops under modern relations of production are developed at the behest of, or at least in collaboration with, multinational food agencies, an oligarchy of enormous companies who use their power to control the pricing of raw materials. The aim of cash cropping is to produce profitable returns on their investments with profitable commodities produced by poorly paid labour. Crops are linked in to a global commercial market and as such are subject to its vicissitudes. Research on the Kenyan coffee-growing region illustrates the health consequences of this:

> Living conditions in coffee growing areas have deteriorated as the fortunes of the crop have diminished. There are many coffee owners who are unable to pay their workers, least of all decent wages. Some of the tasks, such as picking, weeding, spraying and transportation, expose people to pesticides and other chemical substances, snakes' and spiders' bites as well as ergonomic hardships. Besides, many employers do not provide their workers with appropriate personal protective equipment and education on use/handling of chemicals. Trade unions are also too poorly represented in terms of human resources on the ground to make much impact.[22]

To return to WHO's linkage of poverty with high fertility, looked at this way fertility rates are also governed by international commerce. And, of course, the use of child labour spreads beyond the food industry with fashion and technology-based manufacturers being caught in the act of employing children on poverty wages over the recent past.[23]

Private capital also exerts an influence on global health agendas in a very direct way. So-called 'philanthrocapitalism' has come to prominence over the course of the twenty-first century, with largely unaccountable agencies like the Bill and Melinda Gates Foundation (BMGF) and others developing extremely powerful positions on the global health stage. Established in 2000, the BMGF is by far the largest philanthropic organisation in the world. It spends more money on global health than any government other than the US and has a budget bigger and exerts more influence than WHO.[24] BMGF's stated aims are 'harnessing advances in science and technology to reduce health inequalities'.[25] Vaccine distribution and development are a major focus of its operations, with the foundation earmarking over $10 billion over ten years from 2010 to develop and disseminate these. Although important, as history shows, vaccines are, at best, supportive public health tools, historically less effective than improving living conditions, sanitation, safe employment and the like.[26] You might want to pause and reflect here that this model of health improvement driven by medical advance has been discredited since the 1950s. Despite this evidence, BMGF's drugs- and technology-based health focus prevails across the so-called H8, the eight international agencies at the centre of global health initiatives and priorities.[27] In effect, in collaboration with BMGF, the H8 have decided that producing and selling vaccines is more useful than supporting governments to develop good sanitation and clean water, despite decisive historical evidence with regard to health improvements to the contrary.

Among the mechanisms through which BMGF exerts its influence is the PPP model of working which has evolved over the last three decades. As health sociologists Anne-Emmanuelle Birn and Judith Richter argue:

In the early 1990s PPPs of all kinds in a wide array of previously public sector concerns, were promoted as a way of funding and implementing global health initiatives. By the late 1990s, UN agencies had classified a wide range of public–private interactions as 'partnerships' or 'multi-stakeholder initiatives'. Both concepts lump all participants together, erasing key differences in the roles and objectives of those striving for human rights to health and nutrition and those ultimately pursuing their bottom line.[28]

Among other things, these public–private hybrids blur the boundaries between private profit and advancement and public interest, facilitating close relationships between public institutions and business. They support shared decision making between 'stakeholders', enabling BMGF to secure an unprecedented role in global health policymaking, with inadequate public scrutiny or accountability. For example, and to return to the question of nutrition discussed earlier, BMGF and UNICEF set up GAIN, the Global Alliance for Improved Nutrition, in 2002. This PPP has popularised the term 'micronutrient malnutrition' to justify its prime focus on food fortification and supplementation. GAIN argues that 'in an ideal world we would all have access to a wide variety of nutrient rich foods which provide all the vitamins and minerals we need. Unfortunately, for many people, especially in poorer countries, this is often not feasible or affordable'.[29]

These remarks need to be contextualised by the earlier discussion of cash crops, and we might want to join up the dots. Multinational companies, often in collaboration with indigenous governments and supported by their home nation states, buy and redevelop fertile land and compel indigenous populations to work in capital-intensive large-scale farming of cash crops for low wages, contextualising fertility rates. Their global PPP-driven health watchdogs then encourage the belief that health-supporting nutrition levels are not feasible on the diet the populations have been left with and offer them supplements – at a price – to address this, meanwhile positing as a long-term problem the 'high fertility' rates upon which their access to cheap labour depends.

This PPP blurring informs WHO long-term strategies. Central to *Closing the Gap*'s strategies are developing broad partnerships, what the document terms a 'plurality of actors across the field – global institutions and agencies, governments (national and local), civil society, research and academic communities and the private sector'.[30] Health is seen throughout the document as achievable through a coming together of public and private bodies. It is a global version of the purchaser–provider relationships pioneered in local authorities in the UK and US during the 1980s and 1990s. This model means governments and international bodies like WHO buy in the services of or subcontract services out to private health businesses and agencies. The general approach of WHO to working with private health capital was set out in 1998 by the then director general: 'When public and private sectors combine intellectual and other resources more can be achieved'.[31] The growth in consultancy in the international health industry has grown exponentially since the early 2000s when, in a phrase coined by Allan Brandt, 'AIDS invented Global Health'. HIV triggered important new commitments in the funding of healthcare, particularly in developing countries. With the widening recognition of HIV's potential effect on the economic and social development in resource-poor regions, HIV spurred substantial increases in funding from sources such as the World Bank. Given the growing concern in the United Nations and elsewhere that the epidemic posed an important risk to global 'security', new funding was made available from donor countries, ultimately resulting in the establishment of the Global Fund to Fight AIDS, Tuberculosis and Malaria. In 2003, the US Emergency Plan for AIDS Relief (PEPFAR) pledged $15 billion over five years. Since PEPFAR's inception, Congress has allocated more than $46 billion for treatment, infrastructure and partnerships, funding access to global public sector policy and governance for US private capital.[32]

Huge amounts of finance became available in this global health industry. Traditional models and public institutions were supplanted by new PPP-driven models. Governments and international agencies like WHO lost control of the global health agenda. The new global health environment also became a wedge with which private capital could enter new, health-related markets. For example, the giant US management consulting company, McKinsey, recognised in the 'high-aspiration foundations and new global entities ... large, complex entities that are servable by the Firm'. Providing advice to 'governments around the world the same way [as to] corporate clients' enabled private companies to dominate global health agendas.[33]

WHO's partnership approach, outlined in *Closing the Gap*, continues this PPP-based approach, embedding it in their agendas on the basis of the assumption that there are market-based solutions. As Chapter 3 showed, the US medical–industrial complex is very excited about the prospects of this with its 'rising billions' concept. Consultancy, with its focus on short-term solutions, efficiency gains and problem fixing to a budget and for profit, collapses human health and development into an exercise in political economy.

The US, as the primary source of funding for international bodies like the United Nations and WHO, played a major role in establishing the principle that more powerful HICs had a right to intervene in the policies and processes of other countries' governments. Interventions around population control have been a particularly useful tool for US imperialist pretensions for many decades.

Through the 1950s and 1960s aid to LMICs became dependent on a country proving its intent to control their population through appropriate family planning and fertility control measures because, as the World Bank stated in 1968, 'Family planning programmes are less costly than conventional development projects ... [and] yield very high economic returns'.[34] Then president of the World Bank, Robert McNamara put the political relevance of population control even more starkly a year later when he said, 'Are we to solve this problem [overpopulation] by famine? Are we to solve it by riot, by insurrection, by the violence that desperately starving men can be driven to?'[35] There clearly are, and always have been, political motivations driving international bodies and aid agencies like WHO and many others, seeking to intervene in the affairs of LMICs with population control as a stated aim. We might even think that McNamara was more concerned with ensuring a peaceful (and pliant?) population than he was with health.

This chapter has outlined some of the problems international bodies like WHO face in the practical application of the social determinant of health and other health-related principals it espouses. Some of these are to do with faulty and thoroughly outdated theory, in particular with regard to links between fertility rates and poverty. Some of these are to do with the realpolitik of international health agendas, which are being ceded to 'philanthrocapitalism'. The first concern for these profit-oriented organisations is to make populations fit for the exploitative processes through which profits are generated, thus they offer solutions that are in fact the root causes of the problem.

10

The National Health Service: A Revolution Half Made?

The establishment of the NHS is regarded as a high point of British social democracy, representing as it did the outcome of a period of wartime collaboration between social, political and medical elites with organised labour in the guise of the Trades Union Congress (TUC) and the wartime Labour Party. The journey to the 'Appointed Day' is rooted in social and political developments during the interwar years.

The NHS is cherished by people across the political spectrum in British politics. But what is it about the NHS that is so special? Having developed an analysis of how class struggle, mass movements and social and political upheaval on a mass scale influence the social contexts and social determinants of our health, this chapter develops an analysis of the NHS and its coming into being to analyse where this famed institution fits into the health picture. It details the social, economic and political backdrop to general aspirations in the UK for a health service provided centrally by the state. It looks at how the interwar years prepared British society for the change in expectations and delivery of state health provision, and how and why the pace of that process of change accelerated massively during the war years. Finally, the chapter looks at the passing into law of the NHS after the war, with a reformist Labour government bought to power with the biggest working majority in the history of British politics. I finish with a critical examination of the nature of the healthcare service Bevan and his colleagues negotiated and ask, was the NHS a revolution half made?

From the moment of its inception the NHS suffered from financial and governance issues. In 1952, four years after the its creation, one shilling charges for prescriptions and a £1 charge for dental treatment were introduced as the demand for free healthcare outstripped the resources initially allocated. In February 1957 a Royal Commission was set up to consider doctors' pay as a result of medical practitioners' disaffection with their new employment contracts. A year earlier the Guillebaud Report[1] on the financial efficiency of the NHS put the higher than expected costs of healthcare down to teething problems and called for more public funding for hospital modernisation, suggesting £30 million worth of investment per year for seven years from 1958 onwards, as well as recommending increases for community care. Neither of these goals was achieved. Standards of NHS care for disabled people, and especially those in the long-stay institutions established during the latter part of the nineteenth century for people with learning disabilities and those for people with mental health problems, hardly improved at all as a result of the paucity of funding for them following the 1948 National Health Service Act. Throughout its 70-year history financial and governance worries have bedevilled the NHS.

A left-of-centre critique of British medical provision first found voice in the work of Fabian pioneers Sidney and Beatrice Webb. Their contribution to a 1907 Royal Commission on the Poor Law, to that point the nearest to healthcare provision the UK had come, was to submit what became known as the 'Minority Report', later developed and published as *The State and the Doctor*.[2] In this they critiqued what the Royal Commission conceded was a 'state of chaos and confusion' among competing provision from private, Poor Law and Public Health Authority health services.[3] The Webbs argued for a 'unified medical service', a theme which became broadened out and commonly expressed across the left during the interwar years. For the Webbs in this pre-World War I context it simply meant a bringing together of the two categories of medical practitioners who served the working class and poor – Poor Law and Public Health Authority doctors. The commission's solution was the National Health Insurance Act (1911), a state-led health intervention utilising the private sector. The Act provided sickness benefits and access to a private clinician for working people by way of insurance, with contributions paid by workers and topped up by government. Doctors also benefited and were able to secure a more reliable source of income through building up a 'panel' of patients. These 'panel doctor' arrangements persisted until World War II.

A backdrop to these developments and, as we have seen, a constant theme in healthcare and health improvements, was the intensity of industrial unrest in the run up to World War I. Health, and in particular industrial health and safety, were prominent issues among working-class activists and a constant concern for the working class from its birth. In the UK, what has become known as the Great Labour Unrest (1910–14) were years of intense industrial struggle, with over ten million strike days 'lost' annually.[4] Trade union membership rose from 2.1 million to over 4.1 million over the period,[5] a growth unparalleled since the unrest of 1871–3 and the 'new unionism' of 1889–91. As Holton argues, however, this period of strike action was characterised by a particularly 'high degree of aggressive, sometimes violent and often unofficial industrial militancy'.[6] In each of the major strikes during that period – in transport, the mines, engineering, the docks and elsewhere – workers consistently raised demands with regard to their conditions of employment and health more generally. In other words, underpinning the National Insurance Act of 1911 was the widespread and intense industrial struggle of the period.

Poor Law hospitals dominated the healthcare provision for poorer people in the interwar years, only changing in 1929 with the Local Government Act when hospital responsibilities were transferred from the often-hated Poor Law guardians to local authorities. Poor Law hospitals were administered by PACs. In effect these were little more than a reincarnation of the old Boards of Guardians which had run what passed for welfare provision since the 1870s. The Poor Law, or PAC hospitals were converted workhouses, many of which survived beyond the creation of the NHS and on into the twenty-first century. Alongside them was the voluntary healthcare sector whose hospitals accounted for about a quarter of all available hospital beds. A group of over a thousand, the voluntary hospitals ranged from the long-established and large teaching hospitals to small and ill-equipped local provision. A report of 1938 looking at hospitals in Sheffield and the east Midlands found that short-stay cases, typically of less than 20 days, was the norm in voluntary hospitals. Nearly all chronic cases were passed to the PAC hospitals in conditions of 'bare overcrowded, large wards, with cheerless, uncomfortable day rooms and primitive facilities', with patient to staff ratios often exceeding 60 to 1. With parallels to today, voluntary sector healthcare providers faced increasing financial problems. The standards of care available in these mostly small units with limited human and technological resources were low. Successive governments since the early 1920s had not financially supported them. As a result, many offered wards of a better standard for fee-paying patients, establishing a two-tier system.

The larger, teaching hospitals faired better, with access to substantial private endowments and being able to charge higher fees of their wealthier patients, though they also faced deep financial difficulties. Poor Law hospitals were in a terrible state of repair and councils were expected to fund refurbishments. In practice, many local authorities avoided this, instead often paying for acute patients to be sent to city hospitals, while leaving their institutions for older and chronically sick patients virtually untouched in poor repair.[7]

In terms of GP services a district medical officer system was in force which Poor Law authorities controlled. Local authorities contracted a GP to give medical treatment to the uninsured poor. Although GPs could decide whether or not to treat emergency cases the local authority decided on eligibility for free treatment. Even as 'panel' doctors they had little incentive to offer more than a very basic service since they often had to supply medicines and even bandages themselves.[8] In response to this inadequate patchwork of healthcare provision, by 1930 the Socialist Medical Association (SMA) was arguing for: 'A unified state medical service, universal in scope and free to all; served by a full-time salaried staff, including medical practitioners; organised around the key institution of the health centre; emphasising preventative rather than curative medicine; and under democratic control, primarily at local level.'[9]

In the political debates on health in the 1930s, up to and through the war period, political opinion and forces were arranged as follows. Occupying the left position was the SMA, at times with the relatively small Communist Party of Great Britain in tow, and known to us today as the Socialist Health Alliance. To the right, most often, was the collection of health professional bodies, including the Royal Society of Physicians, the BMA and others, usually supported by Conservative Party governments and individuals. Somewhere in the middle was a broad Liberal-Labour consensus, often with ideas and ideologies driven at a conceptual level by Fabianism (Beveridge, for example – he of the founding statement of the welfare state – was a Fabian, schooled by the Webbs, originally a member of the Labour Party and later becoming a Liberal). The voice of organised labour was represented most powerfully by the TUC. Pre-war, the TUC had largely been content to allow the Fabianism which at the time informed both right-wing Labour and Liberal party opinion and policy, to address issues of health. All parties changed their views on healthcare provision from the 1930s through to the Appointed Day in

1948, during a period of economic and political crisis and ideological flux, with some elements of the Liberal-Labour consensus in the middle vacillating rapidly between positions.

In 1932, the director of the London School of Economics and future chairman of the Labour Party, Harold Laski, was asking whether: 'evolutionary socialism [had] deceived itself in believing that it can establish itself by peaceful means within the ambit of the capitalist system'.[10] In its own version of a future health service, and consciously drawing on the ideas of the SMA, the Labour Party Manifesto of 1934 said:

(1)   The nation needs a medical service planned as a whole
(2)   It must be preventive as well as curative; and neither paid private doctoring nor National Health Insurance can deal adequately with the prevention of ill health
(3)   The service must be complete and it must be open to all, so that poverty shall be no bar to health
(4)   It must be efficient and up to date providing for team work – and only the community can achieve this by a planned disposition of hospitals and doctors, etc.
(5)   It must offer a fair deal to doctor and patient alike and only a system of whole time, salaried and pensionable doctoring will do.[11]

In the mid-1930s the Labour Party had begun to base its ideas of a health service on a radical critique of what was then available. At this point Labour championed a future health service based on a preventative as well as curative approach, based in democratically controlled local health centres staffed by salaried professionals – a service planned, funded and run by central government. They recognised that health systems then in existence did not address the needs of the vast majority of the population, and as such were unreliable in providing a fit and healthy workforce for British capital. Neither did it suit the needs of most doctors in general practice. For a well-established GP in a wealthy area life was good. For a young 'Panel' doctor in a poorer area, dependent on National Health Insurance patients or those accessing healthcare via the numerous local health clubs established in most working-class areas, income was low and unpredictable. As historian Pat Thane concludes: 'Just as it had become clear by 1914 that the free market could meet neither the need nor, by 1918, the demand for housing so in the 1930s it was becoming evident that it could meet neither the need nor demand for healthcare.'[12]

It wasn't only the SMA and the Labour Party that recognised something radical needed doing. In 1937 the Conservative Party's Harold Macmillan launched his 'Middle Way',[13] calling for state funding to support private sector investment across a range of industries, including healthcare. Macmillan insisted that trade unions were an essential part of this process and suggested that trade union membership should become compulsory. Suffice to say his ideas were not accepted by the Conservative government of the time, but they do give an idea of this growing reforming centre, taking shape around Liberals such as Beveridge, the Fabian Society and radical Conservatism, articulating the need for far-reaching change in health and welfare provision. As a contemporary report of the time stated: 'It was only with the greatest difficulty that anyone could be persuaded to regard the chaotic and anachronistic structure of medical practice and hospital services as of any real importance to the nation.'[14]

By the time war came, it was accepted across the political spectrum that no return to old systems of healthcare was possible. The debate was about what types of new systems should be adopted. The intensity and pace of this debate increased tenfold as war began. At the beginning of the war health services consisted of:

A rigid and conservative institution ... a multiplicity of individual-istic voluntary hospitals, ranging from the great teaching hospitals to the small, debt-ridden institutions sometimes over-proud of their operating theatres but often short of surgical specialists ... on the other hand, there were the local authority hospitals, tied to out-worn boundaries, receivers of all the unwanted and uninteresting 'chronic' cases, still flavoured with the stigma of the poor law, and often badly equipped and accommodated in large, prison-like buildings.[15]

At the very beginning of hostilities in 1939, informed by the critiques which had evolved during the 1930s, the Emergency Medical Service (EMS) was set up. This was a national health service in all but name. It was centrally planned, administered and financed, bringing together the interwar strands of provision under the control of the Ministry of Health. Britain was divided into regions. Under the EMS, hospitals in the centres

of towns initially received war casualties and patients with major problems, treated them, then transferred them to base hospitals for further
treatment and recuperation. Originally the categories of patients to treat
were restricted, with Service casualties, sick Civil Defence workers, essential war workers and others treated preferentially, but it soon became
obvious that these restrictions were counterproductive and ethically
unacceptable to healthcare staff. Indeed, from the beginning, medical
staff found ways of treating any and all patients with serious illness in
the new, state-run provision.[16] Doctors and nurses were employed by the
state and salaried from the beginning, often at higher rates than before
the war.[17] Personnel and equipment were pooled across hospitals, initiating a collective approach to and distribution of essential resources.
Despite many small and large voluntary hospitals continuing to be selec-
tive of patients in bringing together services under state control, the EMS
clearly demonstrated the advantages of centralised planning and control
of resources. Local authorities took control of running the new systems,
administering local provision and liaising between regions. A free,
needs-led, centrally planned and run service with a salaried staff was
largely in place from 1939, realising much of the vision of the SMA, and
indeed the 1934 Labour Party Manifesto. Many from the Royal Society
of Physicians, along with elements of the BMA and their supporters in
the corridors of power, continued to oppose any change.

Again, as I have shown, underlying long-term developments in healthcare was the activity and organisation of working people. Labour
organisation grew during the war, with trade union membership
climbing from 6.3 million members in the late 1930s to 8.8 million by
1946. Walter Citrine, the relatively moderate leader of the TUC at the
time, argued that 'In wartime there was no room for the unorganised
person'.[18] He demanded that the government should ensure that any
industrial agreements between employers and unions should be
applicable across the industry as a whole. The TUC demanded that
hitherto 'unorganised industries' should be included in 'the principles of
collective bargaining' and generally saw the war, with its need for a disci-
plined, productive workforce engaged in support of the British military
war machine, as an opportunity to widen and deepen the political
strength and influence of trade unions. A number of committees and
other bodies were subsequently – and very quickly – established, giving
institutionalised influence to the TUC, including the first National

Advisory Council to the Minister of Labour, which was established in October 1939.

War put rank-and-file workers in a strong position to address long-held grievances with regard to conditions of employment and wage rates. During the first few months of the war, there were over 900 strikes, almost all of them very short and illegal. The number of strikes increased each year until 1944, almost half of them in support of wage demands and the remainder against deteriorations in workplace conditions. In 1943 there were two major stoppages: one was a strike of 12,000 bus drivers and conductors and the other of dockers in Liverpool and Birkenhead. The year 1944 marked the peak of wartime strike action with over 2,000 stoppages involving the loss of 3,714,000 days' production.[19] Shipbuilding unions won an increase of 10p a week for time workers and 4 per cent for piece workers. Engineers and foundry workers and the Confederation of Shipbuilding and Engineering unions won an extra 25p per week, causing other shipbuilding unions to win an extra 25p per week 'war bonus'. Engineering unions secured an additional 15p per week, on top of the above increases for women over 18 to compensate for the lower rates they had traditionally been paid. Steelworkers, seamen, railway workers and miners all secured substantial wage increases at the very beginning of the war.[20] Nearly all trade boards raised their statutory wage rates at some time during the first eight months of war. In 1940 agricultural workers, long plagued by low pay and seasonal work, won a national minimum wage for men for the first time in their history. Many thousands of women were recruited to wartime industry. In 1940, the engineering federation agreed that women would receive equal pay after 32 weeks in post. Over 20,000 women were employed at the Rolls Royce Hillington site in Glasgow. Rolls Royce evaded the 1940 equal pay formula and were challenged by the AEU in 1943. They settled, but 16,000 women (and some men) refused to accept the deal and walked out for over a week. They won a new agreement which guaranteed the rate for the job, regardless of who was operating the equipment.[21]

Overall, over the six years of war, taking into account the potential for overtime payments, average wages rose by around 76 per cent. Price inflation was high and taxation rose throughout the war, but still workers moved to a higher-wage outlook within the context of secure employment.[22] Wage rises and the spread of collective bargaining saw a substantial increase in union membership during the war, with the figure rising from 6.3 million to 8.8 million by 1946. There were more strike days between 1939 and 1946 than throughout the 1930s.[23]

All of this is indicative of a real shift in the balance of class forces during the period of hostilities, as the needs of the British war machine grew and available labour was depleted. As illustrated by higher levels of organisation, strike action and wage rises, workers expressed their new-found confidence after the long period of retreat of the 1930s. This, I would argue, is the key determinant of the creation of the welfare state, with the NHS at its centre post-war. In this sense, the NHS is the embodiment of the collective strength and will of working people and a core reason why it continues to be cherished and defended by so many millions of us. Working people and their union organisations and leaders took on leading roles in the collective struggle to defeat fascism. Workers felt empowered and expressed that materially, winning better, healthier working conditions and pay, and having a decisive, if not the decisive, voice in deciding how UK society should be structured during wartime. There was an expectation that this should continue afterwards. It was not the rhetorical skills of the famed Churchill but the strength of collective organisation of working people themselves that sustained the UK population through war. Churchill's much feted 'We will fight them on the beaches' speech wasn't even recorded until 1949, let alone broadcast to the nation. It was not heard by British people in any numbers until a recording of it was released by Decca in 1964. Such is the myth-making of bourgeois history.

The Labour Party reaped the benefits of this working-class confidence in the General Election of 1945 when, as we know, the Labour Party won its first parliamentary majority, with the biggest swing of votes – 10.7 per cent – in the history of British politics. The party had a majority of 146 seats, over 60 per cent of the seats in Parliament. Here was the opportunity in terms of health provision to further develop the gains made during the war and to work towards the vision of a national health service that the Labour Party itself had expressed barely ten years before with its calls for a service 'planned as a whole', 'preventive as well as curative', a service 'centred on health centres that only the community can achieve' with a 'salaried and pensionable' staff of doctors. What eventually passed into law as the NHS in 1948 was somewhat different to this, and this final section of the chapter asks why.

The ideological driving force of a centrally planned and administered, preventative health service had from the beginning been the SMA. Their influence, both on public debate and parliamentary politics specifically, had been greatly enhanced by their alliance with the TUC. Early on the SMA had enjoyed the ear of Citrine and others in the leadership of the TUC and through this had been able to set the pace in terms of a programme of change in health provision. This privileged access came to a crashing halt as war neared its end and the possibility of a TUC-backed Labour Party in power began to look a possibility. In 1944 the Conservative Minister of Health Henry Willink signed off a White Paper, 'A National Service for Health'. In a move away from themes that had dominated discussion of a future health service during the war, the paper did not discuss building a unified, centrally controlled system, although a limited role for health centres was envisaged. The issue of democratic local control of provision (something that had actually developed during wartime as many local authorities took control of health services in their area) was fudged, with vague proposals for joint authority duties to plan services through contracting out of services. Nor was the principal of the state paying a salaried medical staff in hospitals and local practice discussed, a key demand of the SMA supported by the TUC and the Labour Party, and voted for by the Medical Practitioners' Union, in the early 1940s. As they had been largely throughout, the BMA were against even the limited reforms of this White Paper. The TUC were largely silent on these key issues. At this time the TUC felt any future NHS needed the 'goodwill of the profession'.[24] Allies previously, as the end of war approached the TUC actively undermined the left wing of the debate expressed by the SMA, and in 1945 the TUC declined their annual invitation to the SMA's conference, stating that 'the invitation should not be accepted in view of the fact that the General Council were acting on behalf of all of its affiliated organisations'.[25] The Fabians, the reformist organisation which had inspired Beveridge, also attacked the SMA. In their document, 'The Principles of a Comprehensive Health Service' of 1943, the Fabians accused the SMA of proposing an 'urban conception' of a health service, centred on health centres and controlled by local authorities which, according to the Fabians, were 'bourgeois and at worst, almost fascist'.[26] As the real possibility of government approached, both the TUC and the ideological leadership of the Labour Party, the Fabians, attacked the left and moved closer to a position from which they could collaborate with the vested interests of pre-war arrangements. It is within this context of a retreat from the more radical, left-wing ideas that we need to consider Health Minister Aneurin Bevan's period of negotiations which led to the final formulations of the health service passed into law on the Appointed Day, 5 July 1948.

In effect, Bevan negotiated the future shape of a national health service which had already been in existence since the beginning of the war. His final settlement was in a form that continued largely to satisfy the demands of a very well-organised and combative working class. However, crucially, it was also in a form that reintegrated to their great satisfaction ancient health hierarchies and vested interests that had been largely put aside during the war to the benefit of a national, collective system of healthcare. At this level of governance and preference Bevan's 'compromises' maintained the dominance of biomedical hierarchy. Bevan's first draft of the proposals was circulated in 1946. As far as the hospital service was concerned, the new proposals went a long way to meet the desires of the medical profession and the voluntary hospital movement. The doctors had feared a salaried service, with loss of clinical freedom. Bevan's plan avoided this. The voluntary hospitals had looked for a way to preserve their independence, though dependent on public funds. They had therefore opposed local authority control, seeking instead partnership on a management body alongside the representatives of local government. This was accepted by Bevan. A regional solution was reached, with the powerful university hospitals given special privileges. Indeed, the British Hospitals Association, representing the 'vested interests' in the Royal Society and BMA, wrote to Bevan that 'so far as concerns the arrangements for the general administration and financing of the service we are satisfied that a substantial measure of common ground is already in sight'.[27]

The London voluntary hospitals were against what they regarded as the 'seizure' of the hospitals by the state, even though that meant state funded financial security along with the various endowments and trust funds that went with that. Sir Bernard Docker of the British Hospitals Association expressed this stating that in terms of 'the crucial question of ownership ... the present proposals bear no relation to our accumulated experience or to the historical evidence of achievement of voluntary as compared to other hospitals'.[28] The highly influential health think tank, the King's Fund, supported this view, and Bevan accepted the voluntary hospitals' 'rights' to keep their own funds within a state provided service.

Sir George Aylwen (London Voluntary Hospitals Committee and St Bartholomew's) wrote to Bevan asking whether existing boards and board members could be retained. Bevan replied that the new boards would be designed to include the more valuable members of the old ones and that he intended 'the reconstructed teaching hospitals to enjoy the various endowments vested in them'. And what about historical treasures, the voluntary hospitals asked? Guy's was worried about the fate of 'an almost unique set of Hepplewhite chairs' – would they be snatched away to the Victoria and Albert for the benefit of the nation as a whole? An assurance was given that no such action would be taken. The summary of the Bill confirmed that the endowments of the voluntary teaching hospitals would pass directly to the new boards of governors, which themselves included many of those who had controlled health provision before the war began.[29] The private endowments and positions of authority for pre-war vested interests were almost completely reinstated by Bevan following the collectivised resourcing and management of the wartime EMS. In this very real sense, the 1948 Act was a step backwards from wartime arrangements.

The senior members of the London County Council (LCC), which had taken control of health services during the war, used their influence to contain opposition to Bevan's plans. In April 1946, Lord Latham, leader of London County Council, said that he and his party deplored the taking away of the LCC hospitals and the encroachment upon local government. Only a quarter of the hospitals in the country were voluntary – the remainder were municipal and the government had taken over the voluntary ones during the war. Latham agreed that there could not be two systems, but instead of insisting on maintaining the highly successful EMS arrangements he agreed, in order to placate vested interests, that the LCC would agree with Bevan in ceding control of the new NHS to them.

Most teaching hospitals understood they had much to gain from the NHS. As noted above, many had faced financial ruin pre-war. By 1947 two-thirds of the income of St Thomas's Hospital came from state or local authority sources, and the situation was much the same at Guy's and the other teaching hospitals. While they feared the loss of autonomy associated with 'nationalisation', they regarded 'municipalisation' (control by local authorities) as worse. One of the St Thomas's staff wrote that had the hospital had the power to decide its own fate in a national health service, it could hardly have chosen better than to follow the course laid down for it by Parliament.[30] Post-war Hospital Boards of Governors were comparable in size to pre-war management committees, and similar in membership. The sometimes-substantial endowment moneys of the teaching and voluntary hospitals had been preserved, and the boards were corporate bodies with the power to hold land and property separately from the state. The burden of debt had been lifted and the extent of local autonomy was considerable. In a memorandum sent to all hospital board chairmen, Bevan wrote that he wanted them to feel 'a lively sense of independent responsibility'. Planning would be a process of continuing informal consultation between the board, the university, the teaching hospital and government.

Again, Marx is called to mind quoted here in the context of the aftermath of the 1840 revolutions: 'the feudal dignitaries [became] paid officials'.[31] Following the unravelling of the EMS and its replacement by the NHS, vested interests, with their positions of authority based on feudal positions stretching back to the sixteenth century, were simply incorporated into positions of power and influence in the new NHS bureaucracy.

A further compromise, negotiated by Bevan and Lord Moran, president of the Royal College of Physicians and Winston Churchill's personal doctor, completed the retreat to pre-war systems of preference. Their negotiations enshrined in law the rights of the most senior doctors and consultants to continue to take on private practice while employed by the NHS. Bevan is quoted as saying 'I had to stuff their mouths with gold', in order to win over the traditional 'vested interests' of the medical profession to accept the constraints of working within the new national-ised system.[32] One response to this might be to ask, in the context of the biggest swing to the Labour Party in the history of parliamentary democracy, leaving the party with a massive working majority with which it could achieve anything it cared to, why did it need to bribe any section of society? The party had very clearly been given a mandate by the British electorate to make sweeping changes, and specifically to develop the type of health service that it had helped to popularise during the 1930s and that had at least partially been developed by the EMS during wartime – one that employed a salaried staff, was preventative as well as curative and was democratically based around locally controlled health centres. Instead, the Labour Party chose to compromise with traditional forces and bring into law a service which many at the time saw as a backwards step from the service which had evolved through the war years. Some in the SMA, for example, regarded the service that passed into law as a national 'sickness service'[33] rather than a national health service, because of its focus on provision centred on the large teaching hospitals there were steeped in tradition, the monopolising of resources this model represented and the curative rather than preventative model they practised.

So while we continue to celebrate the advances made and passed into law by the 1948 Act – a comprehensive and universal 'free at the point of delivery' service; the uniting of voluntary and municipal sectors through the takeover of a financially insecure voluntary sector; the abolition of the sale of GP practices – we must also be aware of the missed opportunities and the weaknesses of the system, inherent in it from the beginning.

Perhaps a quote from the brilliant German revolutionary, Rosa Luxembourg, who died 100 years ago from the year of this publication, is relevant here. Discussing differences between social and political forces content with partial reform and those seeking fundamental change, she writes:

He who pronounces himself in favour of legal reforms in place of and as opposed to the conquest of political power and social revolution does not really choose a more tranquil, surer and slower road to the same goal. He chooses a different goal. Instead of taking a stand for the establishment of a new social order, he takes a stand for surface modifications of the old order. [34]

We might understand the NHS in this light as a 'surface modification' of the old order, a step forward won by an organised and combative working class which nonetheless failed to realise the full potential of the historical moment.

11

Conclusion

Health inequality is a central concern for all of us, threatening our own health expectations and outcomes, the health of those around us and of whole populations. Poor diets, lack of affordable housing, increasingly stressful employment and more have created a context in which the majority of us have seen our health needs grow. However, it does not seem to be a major concern for those who govern us and employ us. Employment is becoming more stressful and potentially harmful to health, not less. Food standards are dropping, housing is becoming more expensive. In the name of neoliberalism and austerity the world is becoming a more difficult and less healthy place to live. This book has sketched out the nature of the predicament facing us. In the name of market-focused ideology and chasing future profits, governments the world over press ahead with privatised models of healthcare, many of which have shown themselves to be incapable of providing adequate care. The care systems in the UK and the US attest to this. The dominant health paradigm, long predicated on the false premise that economic growth is the powerhouse of better health, is one centred on health as a commodity, to be bought and sold via increasingly unregulated markets in healthcare provision, drugs and health insurance. In the UK tens of thousands continue to protest and organise to attempt to hold back this market-driven tide, while in the US too populations register their protest. The medical–industrial complex and its influence represents a future that only active resistance can avoid. The increasingly monopolising tendencies of healthcare strides the globe in search of the 'rising billions' that technology can reach in an openly multinational corporate and pernicious philanthrocapitalist guise.

In the materialist and political content that a social determinants of health approach provides us with, we have a means of both understanding where health inequality is rooted and a means to impact upon it. If we understand health inequality as a conglomerate of other factors of more generalised inequality then health improvement opportunities are all around us. A fight for better conditions of work is a fight for better health; a fight for better and more affordable housing to buy or rent is a fight for better health; a fight for better education for our children, for better quality food, against environmental degradation are all means of resisting the broad categories of social and political trends which undermine our health. The immense and growing health inequality research and literature is an ally in this. The work of Dorling, Pickett, Wilkinson, Coburn, Marmot and others has opened to scrutiny elements of social and political life otherwise perniciously undermining our well-being. This book takes issue with the solutions to these problems implied by the use of subjective categories of analysis, but acknowledges and welcomes the major impact this body of work continues to have. *Vital Signs* presents an analysis of health inequalities which does not arise as a result of a system of economic production behaving in unfair and illogical ways, but as a system working in the only way it can, through the process of exploitation at its centre which is thoroughly injurious to human health. Exploitation, the 'normal' modus operandi of capitalism, produces not simply health inequality, based as it is on the fundamental certainty of inequality in the exploitation process where one class seeks to take from another, but a health deficit. Exploitation together with the alienation resulting from it reduces our overall capacity for holistic health.

Where does the struggle to maintain and defend the NHS fit into this? The institution is a bulwark against the incursions of private health capital; the phrase 'free at the point of delivery' is a beacon of resistance and hope that has echoed down its 70-year history. The NHS represents the idea of a community looking after each other, a collective sense of rights and responsibilities to each other earned by our grandparents and great grandparents and some payment for what they sacrificed. It is a representation of historical victories. But it's not only that. The analysis developed in Chapter 10 showed that models other than those that were curative, led by tradition and centred on the big historic teaching hospitals were on offer and indeed debated until late on in the decision-making process. Democratically controlled, preventative models of services based in communities had dominated discussions about the shape of future provision until Bevan signed off the final agreement. We must learn from this and be aware of the fundamental differences between those who want and need something radically new and those who seek compromise with the old, as we defend what we already have.

Vital Signs concludes that to break the ever-tightening stranglehold of the medical–industrial complex and its health as commodity approach, a paradigm shift is required. Only through the general realignment of social and political priorities implicit in major and general struggle, do new ideas emerge. Achieving better health is a collective, political act to do with providing better social and political environments in which good health can flourish and become meaningful beyond the ideological constraints of health as 'the continued capacity to work'. Without going beyond the constraints of a capitalist mode of production – without moving into a society which produces what it needs in different ways other than via exploitation on the basis of different social classes – health improvements will continue to be partial and time-limited. If exploitation infers a health deficit, only developing a society without exploitation can provide social and political contexts in which our full health potentials can be realised.

Notes

Chapter 1

1. Chan, M., Ten years in public health 2007–2017 (13 April 2017), www.who.int/publications/10-year-review/dg-letter/en/.
2. Birn, A., Pillay, Y. and Holtz, T. (2017) *Textbook of Global Health* (4th edition), Oxford University Press, p. 47.
3. Larson, J., The conceptualisation of health, *Medical Care Research and Review*, 56:2, pp. 123–36 (1999).
4. Stokes, J., Definition of terms and concepts applicable to clinical preventive medicine, *Journal of Community Health*, 8, pp. 33–41 (1982).
5. Constitution of WHO: principles (22 July 1946), www.who.int/about/mission/en/.
6. The Ottawa Charter for Health Promotion, First International Conference on Health Promotion, Ottawa, 21 November 1986, www.who.int/health promotion/conferences/previous/ottawa/en/.
7. Gerhardt, U., Models of illness and the theory of society: Parson's contribution to the early history of medical sociology, *International Sociology*, 5:3, pp. 337–55 (1990).
8. See, for example, Giddens, A., *Central Problems in Social Theory*, Palgrave, 1979.
9. See especially Morgan, M., et al., *Sociological Approaches to Health and Medicine*, Croom Helm, 1985; Samson, C. (ed.), *Health Studies: A Critical and Cross-Cultural Reader*, Blackwell, 1999.
10. Antonovsky, A., *Unraveling the Mystery of Health: How People Manage Stress and Stay Well*, Jossey-Bass, 1987.
11. Canguilhem, G. (1989) *The Normal and the Pathological*, Zone Books.
12. Feig, C. and Shah, S., Setting the record straight on WHO funding (November 18 2011), www.foreignaffairs.com/articles/2011–11–18/setting-record-straight-who-funding.
13. Ibid.
14. Pickett, K. and Wilkinson, R. Income inequality and health: A causal review, *Social Science & Medicine*, 128, pp. 316–26 (2015).
15. Wilkinson, R. and Pickett, K. (2010) *The Spirit Level: Why Equality Is Better for Everyone*, Penguin.
16. Wilkinson, R. and Pickett, K. (2018) *The Inner Level: How More Equal Societies Reduce Stress*, Penguin.

17. www.theguardian.com/inequality/2018/sep/18/kate-pickett-richard-wilkinson-mental-wellbeing-inequality-the-spirit-level.

18. WHO (2008), *Closing the Gap in a Generation: Health Equity Through Action on the Social Determinants of Health*, World Health Organisation, https://apps.who.int/iris/bitstream/handle/10665/43943/9789241563703_eng.pdf?sequence=1.

19. Marmot, M., Rose, G., Shipley, M. and Hamilton, P.J., Employment grade and coronary heart disease in British civil servants, *Journal of Epidemiology and Community Health*, 32:4, pp. 244–9 (1978).

20. Marmot, M., Davey Smith, G., Stansfield, S., et al. Health inequalities among British civil servants: the Whitehall II study, *Lancet*, 337:8754, pp. 1387–93 (1991).

21. Marmot, M., *Status Syndrome: How Your Place on the Social Gradient Directly Affects Your Health*, Bloomsbury, 2015.

22. Ibid.

23. Dorling, D. (2018) *Peak Inequality: Britain's Ticking Time Bomb*, Policy.

24. Ibid.

25. Marmot, M. (2010) *Fair Society, Healthy Lives: Strategic View of Health Inequalities in England Post-2010*, Institute of Health Equity.

26. Townsend, P. and Davidson, N. (1983) *Inequalities in Health: The Black Report*, Pelican.

27. Dorling, D. and Pickett, K., Against the organization of misery? The Marmot Review of health inequalities, *Social Science & Medicine*, 71, pp. 1231–33 (2010).

28. Ibid.

29. Townsend, P. and Davidson, N. (1983) *Inequalities in Health: The Black Report*, Pelican.

30. Dorling, D. (2018) *Peak Inequality: Britain's Ticking Time Bomb*, Policy.

31. Tansey, R., The creeping privatisation of healthcare: Problematic EU policies and the corporate lobby push, Corporate Europe Observatory (2 June 2017), https://corporateeurope.org/power-lobbies/2017/06/creeping-privatisation-healthcare.

Chapter 2

1. Watkins, J., Effects of health and social care spending constraints on mortality in England: A time trend analysis, *BMJ Open*, 7:1 (2017), https://bmjopen.bmj.com/content/7/11/e017722.

2. Keshavjee, S. (2014) *Blind Spot: How Neoliberalism Infiltrated Global Health*, University of California Press.

3. Carter, R., Rise in care homes going out of business (26 April 2016), www.communitycare.co.uk/2016/04/26/rise-care-homes-going-business/.

4. Oxfordshire Social Care Provider Conference at Ruskin College, Oxford (April 2017).

5. Jakubowski, E., Healthcare systems in the EU: A comparative study, European Parliament Working Paper, SACO 101 EN (1998).

6. Hobsbawm, E. (1997) *The Age of Revolution: Europe 1789–1848*, Abacus.

7. Health Foundation, NHS spends about EU average as percentage of GDP on health (30 August 2017), www.health.org.uk/chart/chart-nhs-spends-about-eu-average-as-percentage-of-gdp-on-health.

8. Ibid.

9. Ibid.

10. Plimmer, G., Carillion collapse set to cost taxpayer at least £148m, *Financial Times* (7 June 2018).

11. Kings Fund, Attitudes to NHS and social care funding (2012), www.kingsfund.org.uk/projects/time-think-differently/trends-public-attitudes-expectations-nhs-social-care-funding.

12. *Daily Telegraph*, NHS is fifth biggest employer in world (20 March 2012), www.telegraph.co.uk/news/uknews/9155130/NHS-is-fifth-biggest-employer-in-world.html.

13. Anandaciva, S., NHS myth-busters, Kings Fund (20 November 2017), www.kingsfund.org.uk/publications/nhs-myth-busters.

14. Borneo, A., Helm, C. and Russell, J., *Safe and Effective Staffing: Nursing Against the Odds*, RCN Policy Report, 2017.

15. Tansey, R., The creeping privatisation of healthcare: Problematic EU policies and the corporate lobby push, Corporate Europe Observatory (2 June 2017), https://corporateeurope.org/power-lobbies/2017/06/creeping-privatisation-healthcare.

16. Kuhn, T. (2012) *The Structure of Scientific Revolutions*, University of Chicago Press.

17. Robertson, R., Should we be worried about CCG conflicts of interest? Kings Fund (29 September 2015), www.kingsfund.org.uk/blog/2015/09/should-we-be-worried-about-ccg-conflicts-interest.

18. Anandaciva, S., NHS myth-busters, Kings Fund (20 November 2017), www.kingsfund.org.uk/publications/nhs-myth-busters.

19. Forster, K., Patients at 20 NHS hospitals forced to show passports and ID in 'health tourism' crackdown, *The Independent* (17 January 2017), www.independent.co.uk/news/uk/politics/nhs-hospitals-20-forced-show-passports-id-health-tourism-crackdown-healthcare-jeremy-hunt-government-a7530931.html.

20. Baird, B., et al., Understanding pressures in general practice, Kings Fund (May 2016).

21. Neville, S. and Daneshkhu, S., Consumer drugs do not always work for big pharma, *Financial Times* (6 October 2017), www.ft.com/content/2ffe076c-a485-11e7-b797-b61809486fe2.

22. Skills for Care, The state of the adult social care sector and workforce in England (September 2017), www.skillsforcare.org.uk/stateof.

23. Plimmer, G., M&A on the rise in Healthcare Industry, *Financial Times* (22 October 2012), www.ft.com/content/cee3728e-0707-11e2-92ef-00144 feabdco.

24. Ibid.

25. LaingBuisson (2013) *Social Care Services for Younger Adults with Learning Disabilities and Mental Illness: UK Market Report*, www.laingbuisson.com/wp-content/uploads/2016/06/ScLD1_Bro_WEB_1.pdf.

26. Humphries, R., What now for social care? King's Fund (11 December, 2016), www.kingsfund.org.uk/blog/2016/12/what-now-social-care.

27. UK National Advisory Board to the Social Impact Investment Taskforce, *Building a Social Impact Investment Market: The UK Experience* (September, 2014), www.socialimpactinvestment.org/reports/UK%20Advisory%20 Board%20to%20the%20Social%20Investment%20Taskforce%20Report%20 September%202014.pdf.

28. See www.ashoka.org/en/program/social-financial-services.

29. Finn, D. (2009) The welfare market: The role of the private sector in the delivery of benefits and employment services, in Jane Millar (ed.), *Understanding Social Security: Issues for Policy and Practice*, Policy Press.

30. Plimmer, G., M&A on the rise in healthcare industry, *Financial Times* (22 October 2012), www.ft.com/content/cee3728e-0707–11e2–92ef-00144 feabdco.

31. Lakhani, N. and Whittell, R., Who owns the care homes - and why are they so in debt? *The Independent* (5 November 2012), www.independent.co.uk/ news/uk/home-news/who-owns-the-care-homes-and-why-are-they-so-in-debt-8281273.html.

32. Oksman, O., US firms look to capitalise as NHS becomes increasingly privatised, *The Guardian* (8 February 2016), www.theguardian.com/society/ 2016/feb/08/us-firms-look-to-capitalise-as-nhs-becomes-increasingly-privatised.

33. Ibid.

34. Kramer, L., Against big bets, *Stanford Social Innovation Review* (summer 2017), https://ssir.org/articles/entry/against_big_bets.

35. Little, P., From zombie corps to questionable revenue: Trends to watch for as a health care investor, *Forbes* (17 October 2018), www.forbes.com/sites/ forbesfinancecouncil/2018/10/17/from-zombie-corps-to-questionable-revenue-trends-to-watch-for-as-a-health-care-investor/#74f1ac0753b8.

36. Rushe, D., US stock markets drop amid interest rates hike and looming shutdown, *The Guardian* (20 December 2018), www.theguardian.com/ business/2018/dec/20/us-stock-markets-drop-interest-rates-hike-looming-shutdown.

37. Pratley, N., A shocking way to fund UK care homes, *The Guardian* (12 December 2017), www.theguardian.com/business/nils-pratley-on-finance/ 2017/dec/12/a-shocking-way-to-fund-uk-care-homes.

38. Plimmer, G., M&A on the rise in healthcare industry, *Financial Times* (22 October 2012), www.ft.com/content/cee3728e-0707–11e2–92ef-00144 feabdco.

39. Taylor, O., New survey predicts a 'care crash', *Caring UK* (October 2015).

40. Ruddick, G., Union warns £3bn not enough to save care homes from bankruptcy, *The Guardian* (5 February 2016), www.theguardian.com/ society/2016/feb/05/union-warns-3bn-not-enough-to-save-care-homes-from-bankruptcy.

41. LaingBuisson (2013), *Social Care Services for Younger Adults with Learning Disabilities and Mental Illness: UK Market Report*, www.laingbuisson.com/ wp-content/uploads/2016/06/ScLD1_Bro_WEB_1.pdf.

42. Lakhani, N. and Whittell, R. Who owns the care homes - and why are they so in debt? *The Independent* (5 November 2012), www.independent.co.uk/ news/uk/home-news/who-owns-the-care-homes-and-why-are-they-so-in-debt-8281273.html.

43. Watkins, J., et al., Effects of health and social care spending constraints on mortality in England: A time trend analysis, *BMJ Open*, 7:11 (2017), https:// bmjopen.bmj.com/content/7/11/e017722.

44. O'Connor, S., Tetlow, G. and Bounds, A., National living wage rise heaps care costs pressure on councils, *Financial Times* (1 April 2017), www.ft.com/ content/3eac5a0e-1536-11e7-80f4-13e067d5072c.

45. Powell-Cope, G., Nelson, A. and Paterson, E. (2008) Patient care technology and safety, in Hughe, R. (ed.) *Patient Safety and Quality: An Evidence-Based Handbook for Nurses*, Agency for Healthcare Research and Quality.

46. NHS England, Urgent action pledged on over-medication of people with learning disabilities (14 July2015), www.england.nhs.uk/2015/07/urgent-pledge/.

47. Greener, J. (2016) *The Bottom Line: An Ethnography of For-profit Elderly Residential Care*, PhD thesis, University of Nottingham, https://core.ac.uk/ download/pdf/33565448.pdf.

48. Ibid.

49. Atkinson, C., Families of people with learning disabilities say care is a 'national scandal', *BBC News* (16 July 2015), www.bbc.co.uk/news/blogs-ouch-33535335.

50. Manchester University NHS Foundation Trust, *Operational Plan, 2018–19*, https://mft.nhs.uk/app/uploads/2018/10/MFT-Operational-Plan-v0.21.pdf.

51. Ibid.

Chapter 3

1. Ehrenriech, B. and Ehrenriech, J., cited in Healthcare in the US: Understanding the medical industrial complex, p. 107, in People's Health Movement et al., *Global Health Watch 5: An Alternative World Health Report*, 2017.
2. Woolf, S., Failing health in the US, *BMJ* (7 February 2018).
3. Ibid.
4. Cecere, D., New study finds 45,000 deaths annually linked to lack of health coverage, *Harvard Gazette* (17 September2009), http://news.harvard.edu/gazette/story/2009/09/new-study-finds-45000-deaths-annually-linked-to-lack-of-health-coverage/.
5. Mangan, D., Record number of Obamacare sign-ups on HealthCare.gov for 2017 health insurance coverage, *CNBC* (21 December 2016), www.cnbc.com/2016/12/21/record-number-of-obamacare-signups-on-healthcaregov-for-2017-health-insurance-coverage.html.
6. Smith, D., Has Obamacare become a winning issue for Democrats? *The Guardian* (6 November 2018), www.theguardian.com/us-news/2018/nov/05/obamacare-democrats-midterms-elections.
7. Geyman, J., Crisis in U.S. health care: Corporate power still blocks reform, *International Journal of Health Services*, 48:1, pp. 5–27 (2018).
8. Waitzkin, H. (ed.) (2018) *Health Care Under the Knife: Moving Beyond Capitalism for Our Health*, Monthly Review Press.
9. Mueller, L., 6 ways to protect yourself against rising health care costs, *Forbes* (30 June 2016), www.forbes.com/sites/lucymueller/2016/06/30/why-its-smart-to-be-worried-about-rising-health-care-costs/#7b4e664b65d3.
10. Rice, T., Rosenau, P., Unruh, L. and Barnes, A. (2013) *United States of America: Health System Review, European Observatory on Health Systems and Policies*, www.euro.who.int/__data/assets/pdf_file/0019/215155/HiT-United-States-of-America.pdf.
11. Ibid.
12. Ku, L. and Brantley, E., Myths about the Medicaid expansion and the 'able-bodied', *Health Affairs* (6 March 2017), http://healthaffairs.org/blog/2017/03/06/myths-about-the-medicaid-expansion-and-the-able-bodied/.
13. Ibid.
14. Levy, B.S. and Sidel, V.W., Poverty And Health in the United States, Oxford University Press blog (9 November 2013), https://blog.oup.com/2013/11/poverty-public-health-united-states/.
15. Ku, L. and Brantley, E., Myths about the Medicaid expansion and the 'able-bodied', *Health Affairs* (6 March 2017), http://healthaffairs.org/blog/2017/03/06/myths-about-the-medicaid-expansion-and-the-able-bodied/.
16. Centers for Medicare and Medicaid Services (2015) *National Health Expenditures 2015 Highlights*, www.cms.gov/Research-Statistics-Data-and-

Systems/Statistics-Trends-and-Reports/NationalHealthExpendData/ downloads/highlights.pdf.

17. Ibid.

18. Campaign for Sustainable Rx Pricing, The facts about rising prescription drug costs (April 2017), www.csrxp.org/wp-content/uploads/2016/04/ CSRxP_Facts-of-Rising-Rx-Prices.pdf.

19. Burlage, R. and Anderson, M. (2018) The medical industrial complex in the age of financialisation, in Waitzkin, H. (ed.), *Health Care Under the Knife*, Monthly Review Press, pp. 78–9.

20. Morris, M. (2015) 2015 health care providers outlook United States, Deloitte, www2.deloitte.com/content/dam/Deloitte/us/Documents/life-sciences-health-care/us-2015-global-hc-country-reports-011215.pdf.

21. World Bank (2015) *Health Expenditure Data*, http://data.worldbank.org/ indicator/SH.XPD.TOTL.ZS.

22. Singhal, S. and Coe, E., The next imperatives for US healthcare, *McKinsey on Healthcare* (November 2016), https://healthcare.mckinsey.com/next-imperatives-us-healthcare.

23. Doty, M., Edwards, J. and Holmgren, A. Seeing red: Americans driven into debt by medical bills, Commonwealth Fund (August 2005), www. commonwealthfund.org/usr_doc/837_Doty_seeing_red_medical_debt. pdf?section=4039.

24. Donkar, N. (2017) *US Health Service Deals*, PricewaterhouseCoopers, www. pwc.com/us/en/healthcare/publications/assets/pwc-health-services-deals-insights-q4–2016.pdf.

25. For GDP figures go to https://tradingeconomics.com/united-kingdom/gdp.

26. Burlage, R. and Anderson, M. (2018) The medical industrial complex in the age of financialisation, in Waitzkin, H. (ed.), *Health Care Under the Knife*, Monthly Review Press, p. 75.

27. Pierce, M.E., Convergence of the health industry, *International Journal of Health Care Quality Assurance*, 18:1 (2005).

28. James, J.T., A new, evidence-based estimate of patient harms associated with hospital care, *Journal of Patient Safety*, 9:3 (2013).

29. Pierce, M.E., Convergence of the health industry, *International Journal of Health Care Quality Assurance*, 18:1 (2005).

30. Stoakes, U., The rising billions and healthcare's expanding global market, *Forbes* (8 December 2015), www.forbes.com/sites/unitystoakes/2015/12/08/ the-3-trillion-us-healthcare-market-pales-in-comparison-to-the-rising-billions.

31. Darzi, A., The cheap innovations the NHS could take from sub-Saharan Africa, *The Guardian* (27 October 2017), www.theguardian.com/healthcare-network/2017/oct/27/cheap-innovations-nhs-take-sub-saharan-africa.

32. MD, The shocking truth about the nursing shortage in the United States, *Referral MD* (2018), https://getreferralmd.com/2017/12/on-the-verge-of-a-

nursing-shortage/; see also, Fayer, S. and Watson, A., Employment and wages in healthcare occupations, The Bureau of Labor Statistics (December 2015), www.bls.gov/spotlight/2015/employment-and-wages-in-healthcare-occupations/pdf/employment-and-wages-in-healthcare-occupations.pdf.

33. Smith, A. (1776) *Wealth of Nations, Book I, Chapter VI, Of the Component Parts of the Price of Commodities.*
34. Colombo, J. (2017) *The U.S. Healthcare Bubble*, www.thebubblebubble.com/healthcare-bubble/.
35. Howrigon, R., 2017, How health care could crash the US Economy, KevinMD.com (19 January), www.kevinmd.com/blog/2017/01/health-care-crash-u-s-economy.html.
36. Bukharin, N. (1972) *Imperialism and the World Economy*, Merlin.

Chapter 4

1. WHO, Commission on Social Determinants of Health (2008) *Closing the Gap in a Generation: Health Equity Through Action on the Social Determinants of Health*, World Health Organization.
2. Ibid.
3. WHO, World Conference on Social Determinants of Health, Rio political declaration on social determinants of health (2011).
4. WHO, Commission on Social Determinants of Health (2008) *Closing the Gap in a Generation: Health Equity Through Action on the Social Determinants of Health*, World Health Organization, p. 1.
5. Ibid.
6. Ibid.
7. Ibid.
8. Canguilhem, G. (1989) *The Normal and the Pathological*, Zone Books, p. 232; see also Murphy, H., Blood pressure and culture: The contribution of cross-cultural comparisons to psychosomatics, *Psychotherapy and Psychosomatics*, 38:1, pp. 244–55 (1982).
9. See, for example, the body of work of geneticist John Parrington, including (2015) *The Deeper Genome: Why There Is More to the Human Genome than Meets the Eye*, Oxford University Press, where he discusses the theory that our very genetic make up is influenced by cultural environments.
10. Taylor, M., 90% of world's children are breathing toxic air, WHO study finds, *The Guardian* (20 October 2018), www.theguardian.com/environment/2018/oct/29/air-pollution-worlds-children-breathing-toxic-air-who-study-finds.
11. World Health Organization, Air pollution and child health: prescribing clean air, WHO Report (2018), WHO reference number: WHO/CED/PHE/18.01, p. 37.
12. Peoples Health Movement (2017) *Global Health Watch: An Alternative World Health Report*, Zed Books.

13. Ibid., p. 172.

14. Carrington, D., Air pollution 'as bad as smoking in increasing risk of miscarriage', *The Guardian* (11 January 2019), www.theguardian.com/environment/2019/jan/11/air-pollution-as-bad-as-smoking-in-increasing-risk-of-miscarriage.

15. Marshal, J., Ella Kissi-Debrah 'pollution' death: Backing for new inquest, *BBC News* (11 January 2019), www.bbc.co.uk/news/health-46823309.

16. Ibid.

17. De Sa, J., How does housing influence our health? The Health Foundation (31 October 2017), www.health.org.uk/infographic/how-does-housing-influence-our-health.

18. Barker, K. (2004) *Barker Review of Housing Supply – Final Report – Recommendations*, HM Treasury.

19. Ibid., p. 73.

20. NHS, Homeless die 30 years younger than average, NHS (21 December 2011), www.nhs.uk/news/lifestyle-and-exercise/homeless-die-30-years-younger-than-average/.

21. Crisis, *Homelessness Monitor, 2016*, www.crisis.org.uk/ending-homelessness/homelessness-knowledge-hub/homelessness-monitor/england/the-homelessness-monitor-england-2018.

22. Booth, R., Spike in deaths of Oxford rough sleepers rocks community, *The Guardian* (31 January 2019), www.theguardian.com/uk-news/2019/jan/31/spike-in-deaths-of-oxford-rough-sleepers-rocks-community-homeless.

23. UCL Institute of Health (2012) *Economic Downturn*, Institute of Health Equity, pp. 65–9.

24. Ibid., pp. 70–1.

25. Ibid., p. 72.

26. RICS, Residential market survey (July 2017), www.rics.org/uk/news-insight/research/market-surveys/uk-residential-market-survey/.

27. Cribb, J., Hood, A. and Hoyle, J., The decline of homeownership among young adults, Institute for Fiscal Studies (16 February 2018), www.ifs.org.uk/publications/10505.

28. Fitch, C., The relationship between personal debt and mental health: A systematic review, *Mental Health Review Journal*, 16:4, pp. 153–66 (2011), www.emeraldinsight.com/doi/abs/10.1108/13619321111202313.

29. Collinson, P., UK living rooms have shrunk by a third, survey finds, *The Guardian* (8 April 2018), www.theguardian.com/business/2018/apr/08/uk-living-rooms-have-shrunk-by-a-third-survey-finds.

30. King, R., Orloff, M., Virsilas, T. and Pande, T. (2017) *Confronting the Urban Housing Crisis in the Global South: Adequate, Secure, and Affordable Housing*, World Resources Institute, www.wri.org/publication/towards-more-equal-city-confronting-urban-housing-crisis-global-south.

31. Shelter (2005) *Safe and Secure? The Private Rented Sector and Security of Tenure*.

32. King, R., Orloff, M., Virsilas, T. and Pande, T. (2017) *Confronting the Urban Housing Crisis in the Global South: Adequate, Secure, and Affordable Housing*, World Resources Institute, www.wri.org/publication/towards-more-equal-city-confronting-urban-housing-crisis-global-south.

33. Florida, R., The global housing crisis, *Citylab* (11 April 2018), www.citylab.com/equity/2018/04/the-global-housing-crisis/557639/.

34. Woo, R., China house prices to rise faster in 2018 in boost for cooling economy – Reuters poll, Reuters (10 September 2018), https://uk.reuters.com/article/uk-china-property-poll/china-house-prices-to-rise-faster-in-2018-in-boost-for-cooling-economy-reuters-poll-idUKKCN1LQ0TB.

35. Engels, F. (1984) *The Condition of the Working Class*, Lawrence Wishart.

36. Lougheed, K. (2018) *Catching Breath: The Making and Unmaking of Tuberculosis*, Bloomsbury.

37. TBAlert, TB and poverty, www.tbalert.org/about-tb/global-tb-challenges/tb-poverty/.

38. Ibid.

39. Orel, K., Eating yourself to death: The junk food epidemic, *The Real Truth*, https://rcg.org/realtruth/articles/120927–001.html.

40. Ibid.

41. Ibid.

42. Shridhar G., Rajendra N., Murigendra H., Shridevi P., Prasad M., et al. Modern diet and its impact on human health, *Journal of Nutrition and Food Science*, 5:6, p. 430 (2015).

43. Engels, F. (1984) *The Condition of the Working Class*, Lawrence Wishart.

44. Everstine, K., Spink, J. and Kennedy, S., Economically motivated adulteration (EMA) of food: Common characteristics of EMA incidents, *Journal of Food Protection*, 76:4, pp. 723–35 (2013).

45. Pimental, P., Trends and solutions in combating global food fraud, *Food Safety Magazine* (February/March 2014), www.foodsafetymagazine.com/magazine-archive1/februarymarch-2014/trends-and-solutions-in-combating-global-food-fraud/.

46. Morling, A. and McNaughton, R. (2016) *Food Crime Annual Strategic Assessment: A 2016 baseline*, Food Standards Agency.

47. Ibid.

48. Hughes, D., UK eggs declared safe 30 years after salmonella scare, *BBC News* (11 October 2017), www.bbc.co.uk/news/health-41568998.

49. Gossner et al., The melamine incident: Implications for international food and feed safety, *Environmental Health Perspective*, 17:12 (December 2009).

50. Eufic, 2017 Fipronil contaminated eggs: Things to know (23 August 2017), www.eufic.org/en/food-safety/article/eggs-contaminated-with-fipronil-what-do-you-need-to-know.

51. Empson, M. (2017) *Land and Labour: Marxism, Ecology and Human History*, Bookmarks, pp. 124.

52. See, for example, Gunnars, K. (2017) Saturated fat: good or bad? *Healthline*, 22 June; Joseph, M. (2017) 9 reasons saturated fat is good for you: nutrition advance, *Nutrition Advance*, 19 January; Kuzemchak, S. (2012) The truth about saturated fats, *Fitness*, September, www.fitnessmagazine.com/recipes/healthy-eating/nutrition/good-and-bad-fats/; English, N. (2013) Everyone was wrong: saturated fat can be good for you, *Greatist*, 21 November.

53. Feltham, S. (2016) *Healthy Eating Guidelines and Weight Loss Advice For The United Kingdom*, Public Health Collaboration.

54. Blanchard, J., Westminster gravy train: Full list of ex-coalition ministers who are now cashing in with jobs for the boys, *Daily Mirror* (10 January 2016), www.mirror.co.uk/news/uk-news/westminster-gravy-train-full-list-7153687.

55. O'Donnell, J., HHS nominee Tom Price bought stock, then authored bill benefiting company, *USA Today* (2 February 2017), https://eu.usatoday.com/story/news/politics/2017/02/02/hhs-nominee-tom-price-bought-stock-then-authored-bill-benefiting-company/97337838/.

56. Tait, C. (2015) *Hungry for Change: Final Report on the Fabian Commission on Food and Poverty*, Fabian Society.

57. Lewchuk, W., et al., From job strain to employment strain: health effects of precarious employment. *Just Labour* 3 (Autumn 2003), https://justlabour.journals.yorku.ca/index.php/justlabour/article/view/165.

58. Holman, D., Batt, R. and Holtgrewe, U. (2007) *The Global Call Centre Report: International Perspectives on Management and Employment: A Report of the Global Call Centre Research Network*.

59. Sprigg, C., Smith, P. and Jackson, P., Psychosocial risk factors in call centres: An evaluation of work design and well-being, prepared by the University of Sheffield, Health and Safety Laboratory and UMIST for the Health and Safety Executive 2003 Research Report 169.

60. Ibid.

61. Unite the Union (2011) *Health and Safety Guide*.

62. Sprigg, C., Smith, P. and Jackson, P., Psychosocial risk factors in call centres: An evaluation of work design and well-being, prepared by the University of Sheffield, Health and Safety Laboratory and UMIST for the Health and Safety Executive (2003) Research Report 169.

63. Stevenson, D. and Farmer, P. (2017) *Thriving At Work: The Stevenson/Farmer Review of Mental Health and Employers*.

64. Rose, N., Urban social exclusion and mental health of China's rural–urban migrants: A review and call for research, *Health and Place*, 48, pp. 20–30 (2017).

65. ILO, Safety and health at work in China and Mongolia, International Labour Organisation, www.ilo.org/beijing/areas-of-work/safety-and-health-at-work/lang--en/index.htm.

66. ILO, Global report on child labour cites alarming extent of its worst forms, International Labour Organisation, www.ilo.org/global/about-the-ilo/ newsroom/news/WCMS_007784/lang--en/index.htm; see also WHO, Hazardous child labour, www.who.int/occupational_health/topics/ childlabour/en/.

67. HMSO, Children's Employment Commission (1867) *Sixth Report of the Commissioners*, Volume 16, p. 132.

68. ILO (2017) *Child Labour in the Primary Production of Sugar Cane*, International Labour Organisation, p. 21.

Chapter 5

1. Wilkinson, R., Pickett, K. (2009) *The Spirit Level: Why Equality is Better for Everyone*, Bloomsbury, p. 26.

2. Marmot, M., Rose, G., Shipley, M. and Hamilton, P.J., Employment grade and coronary heart disease in British civil servants, *Journal of Epidemiology and Community Health*, 32:4 , pp. 244–9 (1978); Marmot, M., Davey Smith, G., Stansfield, S., et al. Health inequalities among British civil servants: The Whitehall II study, *Lancet*, 337 (8754), pp. 1387–93 (1991).

3. Marmot, M., Rose, G., Shipley, M. and Hamilton, P.J., Employment grade and coronary heart disease in British civil servants, *Journal of Epidemiology and Community Health*, 32:4 , pp. 244–9 (1978).

4. Marmot, M., Davey Smith, G., Stansfield, S., et al. Health inequalities among British civil servants: The Whitehall II study, *Lancet*, 337 (8754), pp. 1387–93 (1991).

5. Ibid.

6. Ibid.

7. Weber, M., Class, status and party, The Middlebury Blog Network, https:// sites.middlebury.edu/individualandthesociety/files/2010/09/Weber-Class-Status-Party.pdf.

8. Giddens, A. (1990) *Central Problems in Social Theory: Action, Structure and Contradictions in Social Analysis*, Palgrave.

9. Humber, L., unpublished MA thesis, University of Leicester (1999).

10. Gould, S.J. (1996) *Full House: The Spread of Excellence from Plato to Darwin*, Harmony Books.

11. Putnam, R., What makes democracy work? *National Civic Review*, 82:2 (1993).

12. See for example Judge, K., Income distribution and life expectancy: A critical appraisal, *British Medical Journal*, 311:12, pp. 82–7 (1995); Gravelle, H., Wildman, J. and Sutton, M. Income, Income inequality and health: What can we learn from aggregate data? *Social Science & Medicine*, 54:5, pp. 77–89 (2001).

13. Coburn, D., Income inequality, social cohesion and the health status of populations: The role of neo-liberalism, *Social Science and Medicine*, 51, pp. 135–46 (2000).

14. Exceptions to this include: Navarro, V., Health and equity in the world in the era of globalization, *International Journal of Health Services*, 29:2 (1999); Muntaner, C. and Lynch, J., Income inequality, social cohesion, and class relations: A critique of Wilkinson's neo-Durkheimian research program, *International Journal of Health Services*, 29:1 (1999); and Scambler, G. and Higgs, P., Stratification, class and health: Class relations and health inequalities in high modernity, *Sociology* (1 May 1999).

15. Wilkinson, R. and Pickett, K. (2010) *The Spirit Level: Why Equality Is Better for Everyone*, Penguin.

16. Ibid.

17. Ibid.

18. See, for example, Coburn, D., Income inequality, welfare, class and health: A comment on Pickett and Wilkinson, *Social Science and Medicine*, 146, pp. 228–32 (2015); Coburn, D., Health inequalities: A response to Scambler, *Sociology of Health and Illness*, 34:1 (2011).

19. Coburn, D., Income inequality, social cohesion and the health status of populations: The role of neo-liberalism, *Social Science and Medicine*, 51, pp. 135–46 (2000).

20. Aaberge, R., et al., Increasing income inequality in the Nordics, *Nordic Economic Policy Review*, Nordic Council of Ministers (2018).

21. Ibid.

22. Merick, R., Minsters broke promise to review pointlessly cruel system for benefit sanctions, MPs say, *The Independent* (6 November 2018), www.independent.co.uk/news/uk/politics/benefit-sanctions-welfare-system-department-work-pensions-conservative-frank-field-a8618766.html.

23. Ibid.

24. Beckfield, J. and Bambra, C., Shorter lives in stingier states: Social policy shortcomings help explain the US mortality disadvantage, *Social Science & Medicine*, 171, pp. 30–8 (2016).

25. Ibid., p. 30.

26. *The Local*, Half of southern Italians at risk of poverty: Report (6 December 2016), www.thelocal.it/20161206/half-of-southern-italians-at-risk-of-poverty-report.

27. Ibid.

Chapter 6

1. Gee, E. and Gutman, G. (eds) (2000) *The Overselling of Population Ageing: Apocalyptic Demography, Intergenerational Challenges and Social Policy*, Oxford University Press.

2. ONS, How do the post-World War baby boom generations compare? (6 March 2018), www.ons.gov.uk/peoplepopulationandcommunity/births deathsandmarriages/ageing/articles/howdothepostworldwarbabyboom generationscompare/2018-03-06.

3. Department of Business, Energy and Industrial Strategy, Trade union membership, 2016, Statistical Bulletin, May 2017.

4. Marmot, M., Life expectancy rises 'grinding to halt', *IEHC News* (19 July 2017), www.ucl.ac.uk/iehc/iehc-news/michael-marmot-life-expectancy.

5. Ibid.

6. Dorling, D., Short cuts: Future life expectancy in the UK, www.dannydorling.org/?p=6219.

7. Marmot, M., Life expectancy rises 'grinding to halt', *IEHC News* (19 July 2017), www.ucl.ac.uk/iehc/iehc-news/michael-marmot-life-expectancy.

8. Ibid.

9. British Nutrition Foundation, How the war changed nutrition: From there to now, www.nutrition.org.uk/nutritioninthenews/wartimefood/warnutrition.html.

10. Ibid.

11. Simkin, J., 1946 School Milk Act, September 1997, https://Spartacus-educational.com/ED1946.htm.

12. Renton, D., Housing: As it is, and as it might be, *International Socialist Journal*, 134 (March 2012).

13. Hennessy, P. (2007) *Having it So Good: Britain in the Fifties*, Penguin.

14. Luxford, C., 'Palaces of the people': Britain's post-war prefabs, *Culture Trip* (28 August 2018), https://theculturetrip.com/europe/united-kingdom/articles/palaces-of-the-people-britains-post-war-prefabs/.

15. Hennessy, P. (2007) *Having it So Good: Britain in the Fifties*, Penguin.

16. Beirne, P. (1977) *Fair Rent and Legal Fiction: Housing Rent Legislation in a Capitalist Society*, Macmillan.

17. Hennessy, P. (2007) *Having it So Good: Britain in the Fifties*, Penguin.

18. Ibid.

19. Hatherley, O., Vienna's Karl Marx Hof: Architecture as politics and ideology, *The Guardian* (27 April 2015), www.theguardian.com/cities/2015/apr/27/vienna-karl-marx-hof-architecture-politics-ideology-history-cities-50-buildings.

20. Goldfinger, E. (1996) *RIBA Drawings Monographs No. 3, Robert Elwall*, www.balfrontower.org/document/15/erno-goldfinger-riba-drawings-monographs-no-3.

21. TUC History online, www.unionhistory.info/timeline/1945_1960_2.php.

22. Ibid.

23. Ibid.

24. Darlington, R., Shop stewards' leadership, left-wing activism and collective workplace union organisation, *Capital & Class*, 26:1, pp. 95–126 (2002).

25. Preston, S., Children and the elderly: Divergent paths for America's dependents, *Demography*, 21:4 (1984).

26. Kotlikoff, L. (1993) *Generational Accounting: Knowing Who Pays, and When, for What we Spend*, Free Press.

27. Callahan, D. (1987) *Setting Limits: Medical Goals in an Ageing Society*, Simon and Schuster.

28. Shelp, E., Our natural lives, *New York Times Book Review* (27 September 1987), www.nytimes.com/1987/09/27/books/our-natural-lives.html.

29. Barry, R. and Bradley, G. (eds) (1991) *Set No Limits: A Rebuttal to David Callahan's Proposal to Limit Healthcare for the Elderly*, University of Illinois Press.

30. See, for example, Ervik, R. (2009) *A Missing Leg of Ageing Policy Ideas: Dependency Ratios, Technology and International Organizations*, International Sociological Association, Research Group 19, Conference on Social Policies: Local Experiments, Travelling Ideas, Montreal, Canada, www.cccg. umontreal.ca/rc19/PDF/Ervik-R_Rc192009.pdf.

31. Gee, E. and Gutman, G. (eds) (2000) The Overselling of Population Ageing: Apocalyptic Demography, Intergenerational Challenges and Social Policy, Oxford University Press.

32. Spijker, J. and MacInnes, J., Population ageing: The timebomb that isn't? *British Medical Journal*, 347 (16 November 2013), www.bmj.com/bmj/section-pdf/749788.

33. McFaul, S., Grandparents who help with childcare at risk of missing out on full state pension—act now to protect it, *MSE News* (18 January 2017), http://tinyurl.com/y7qy2j35.

34. Oxlade, A., World pension ages on the rise: When will you retire? *Schroders* (23 November 2017), www.schroders.com/en/insights/economics/world-pension-ages-on-the-rise-when-will-you-retire/.

35. Roberts, M., The pensions myth: Part one, https://thenextrecession. wordpress.com/2011/12/03/the-pensions-myth-part-one/.

36. Ibid.

37. Dempsey, N., UK defence expenditure, Briefing Paper Number CBP 8175, House of Commons Library (8 November 2018).

38. Hinrich, K., In the wake of the crisis: Pension reforms in eight European countries, ZeS-Working Paper No. 01/2015, www.socium.uni-bremen.de/uploads/News/2015/ZeS-AP_2015_01.pdf).

39. Ibid.

40. Ibid.

41. See, for example, *France24*, French pensioners, health aides kick off Macron reform protests (15 March 2018), www.france24.com/en/20180315-french-pensioners-health-aides-kick-off-macron-reform-protests.

42. Roberts, M., The pensions myth: Part two, https://thenextrecession. wordpress.com/2011/12/03/the-pensions-myth-part-two/.

43. Ibid.
44. Ibid.
45. Courea, E., Pensioner poverty rises as benefits freeze bites, *The Observer* (9 December 2018), www.theguardian.com/society/2018/dec/09/pensioner-poverty-rises-bnefites-freeze.
46. Roberts, M., The pensions myth: Part two, https://thenextrecession.wordpress.com/2011/12/03/the-pensions-myth-part-two/.
47. Ibid.
48. Ibid.
49. Ibid. See also *The Conversation*, Britain's great pension robbery: Why the 'defined benefits' gold standard is a luxury of the past (3 August 2018), http://theconversation.com/britains-great-pension-robbery-why-the-defined-benefits-gold-standard-is-a-luxury-of-the-past-100844.
50. Brayne, C., A life-course approach to prevent dementia, *Bulletin of World Health Organ*, 96:3, pp. 153–4 (1 March 2018), www.ncbi.nlm.nih.gov/pmc/articles/PMC5840636/.
51. Anderson, T., Carol Brayne: A life-course approach to prevent dementia, interview, *Bulletin of the World Health Organ*, 96:3, pp. 153–4 (1 March 2018).
52. Ibid.
53. Ibid.
54. Lo, R., The borderland between normal aging and dementia, *Tzu Chi Medical Journal*, 29(2), pp. 65–71 (April–June 2017), www.ncbi.nlm.nih.gov/pmc/articles/PMC5509201/.
55. Ibid.
56. Ibid.
57. Cohen, L. (1998) *No Aging in India: Alzheimer's, the Bad Family, and Other Modern Things*, University of California Press.

Chapter 7

1. Callinicos, A. (2015) *disClosure: A Journal of Social Theory, Volume 24: Market Failures, Famines, and Crises*, https://uknowledge.uky.edu/cgi/viewcontent.cgi?article=1384&context=disclosure.
2. Foucault, M. (1994) *Birth of the Clinic: An Archaeology of Medical Perception*, Vintage, p. 306.
3. Porter, R. (1997) *The Greatest Benefit to Mankind: A Medical History of Humanity from Antiquity to the Present*, Fontana.
4. The French Revolution: A Revolution in Medicine, Too , Hospital Practice, 12: 11, 1977, Pages 127–38, Published online: 06 Jul 2016.
5. Ibid.
6. Foucault, M. (1994) *Birth of the Clinic: An archaeology of medical perception*, Vintage.

7. The French Revolution: A revolution in medicine, too, *Hospital Practice*, 12:11, pp. 127–38 (1977), published online 6 July 2016.

8. Foucault, M. (1994) *Birth of the Clinic: An Archaeology of Medical Perception*, Vintage.

9. Cantin, Projet de reform adresse a laAssemblee Nationale, cited in ibid., p. 28.

10. Foucault, M. (1994) *Birth of the Clinic: An Archaeology of Medical Perception*, Vintage.

11. The French Revolution: A revolution in medicine, too, *Hospital Practice*, 12:11, pp. 127–38 (1977), published online 6 July 2016.

12. Bacher, De la medicine consideree politiquement, cited in Foucault, M. (1994) *Birth of the Clinic: An Archaeology of Medical Perception*, Vintage, p. 31.

13. Foucault, M. (1994) *Birth of the Clinic: An Archaeology of Medical Perception*, Vintage.

14. Lange, S. and Lu, E., The medical gaze: What do Foucault and the French Revolution have to do with modern medicine? *In-Training* (5 February 2014), http://in-training.org/medical-gaze-4170.

15. Foucault, M. (1994) *Birth of the Clinic: An Archaeology of Medical Perception*, Vintage.

16. Ibid.

17. Labisch, A., Doctors, workers and the scientific cosmology of the industrial world: The social construction of 'health' and the 'homo hygienicus', *Journal of Contemporary History*, 20: 4, pp. 599–615 (1985).

18. Ibid.

19. Ibid., p. 599.

20. Ibid., p. 600.

21. Ibid., p. 600.

22. Ibid.

23. See, for example, Maki, J., Kojma, H., Sakagami, H. and Kuwada, M., European traditional healers persecuted as witches and Kenyan traditional doctors, *Yakushigaku Zasshi*, 34(2), pp. 100–1 (1999), www.ncbi.nlm.nih.gov/pubmed/11624341.

24. Labisch, A., Doctors, workers and the scientific cosmology of the industrial world: The social construction of 'health' and the 'homo hygienicus', *Journal of Contemporary History*, 20: 4, pp. 599–615 (1985).

25. Illich, I. (1976) *Limits to Medicine: Medical Nemesis – The Expropriation of Health*, Pantheon Books, p. 42.

26. NHS, Why we should sit less, www.nhs.uk/live-well/exercise/why-sitting-too-much-is-bad-for-us/.

27. Windsor-Shellard, B., Suicide by occupation, England: 2011 to 2015, Office for National Statistics (17 March 2017), www.ons.gov.uk/peoplepopulation andcommunity/birthsdeathsandmarriages/deaths/articles/suicideby

occupation/england2011to2015#suicide-by-occupation-among-males; https://metro.co.uk/2018/09/03/suicide-rate-rises-in-uk-doctors-and-women-are-more-likely-to-kill-themselves-7907478/.

28. Kekatos, M., Suicide rate of doctors is the highest of any profession and double that of the general population, study finds, *Daily Mail* (1 June 2018), www.dailymail.co.uk/health/article-5792735/Suicide-rate-doctors-highest-profession-DOUBLE-general-population.html.

29. McKay, A. and Majeed, A., Junior doctors in England strike for first time in forty years, *The Journal of Ambulatory Care Management*, 39:2, pp. 178–81 (1 April 2016).

30. Adeline, unpublished thesis, Ruskin College, Oxford (2018).

31. Ibid.

32. Kuhn, T. (2012) *The Structure of Scientific Revolutions*, University of Chicago Press. p. 43.

33. Porter, R. (1997) *The Greatest Benefit to Mankind: A Medical History of Humanity from Antiquity to the Present*, Fontana.

34. www.britannica.com/topic/Natural-and-Political-Observations-Made-Upon-the-Bills-of-Mortality.

35. Porter, R. (1997) *The Greatest Benefit to Mankind: A Medical History of Humanity from Antiquity to the Present*, Fontana, p. 229.

36. Ibid., p. 229.

37. Ibid., p. 230.

38. Foucault, M. (1994) *Birth of the Clinic: An Archaeology of Medical Perception*, Vintage.

39. Sydenham, T., *The Works of Thomas Sydenham*, 2 vols, Latham, R. (ed.), Sydenham Society, 1848, vol. 1, pp. 20–1.

40. Sanchez-Gonzalez, Medicine in John Locke's philosophy, *Journal of Medicine and Philosophy*, 15:6, pp. 675–9 (December 1990).

41. Aspelin, G., Locke and Sydenham, *Theoria*, 15, pp. 29–37 (1949).

42. Laski, H. (2015) *Communism*, Routledge, p. 234.

43. Newsholme, A. and Kingsbury, J. (1934) *Red Medicine: Socialised Health in Soviet Russia*, Heinemann.

44. Ibid., p. 211.

45. Carrell, S., Students from wealthy backgrounds dominate medical schools, *The Guardian* (22 January 2016), www.theguardian.com/society/2016/jan/22/medical-school-students-wealthy-backgrounds.

46. Bukharin, N. (1972) *Imperialism and the World Economy*, Merlin.

47. Carr, E. (1979) *The Russian Revolution: From Lenin to Stalin 1917–1929*, Macmillan, p. 196.

48. Semashko, N., The work of the public health authorities in Soviet Russia, *The Communist Review*, 4:2 (June 1923).

49. Cited in Petegorsky, D. (1995) *Left-Wing Democracy in the English Civil War: Gerrard Winstanley and the Digger Movement*, Alan Sutton Publishing.

50. Kuhn, T. (2012) *The Structure of Scientific Revolutions*, University of Chicago Press, p. 34.

51. Foucault, M. (1994) *Birth of the Clinic: An Archaeology of Medical Perception*, Vintage.

52. Tawney, R., cited in Petegorsky, D. (1995) *Left-Wing Democracy in the English Civil War: Gerrard Winstanley and the Digger Movement*, Alan Sutton Publishing, p. 22.

Chapter 8

1. Chesnais, J.-C. (1992) *The Demographic Transition: Stages, Patterns, and Economic Implications*, Oxford University Press; see also *Sociology Discussion*, The theory of demographic transition, www.sociologydiscussion.com/demography/population-demography/the-theory-of-demographic-transition-with-criticisms/3096.

2. Bynum, B., The McKeown thesis, *The Lancet*, Perspectives, The Art of Medicine, 371:9613, pp. 644–5 (February 23 2008).

3. Porter, R. (1997) *The Greatest Benefit to Mankind: A Medical History of Humanity from Antiquity to the Present*, Fontana.

4. Ibid.

5. McKeown, T. cited in Szreter, S. (2007) *Health and Wealth: Studies in History and Policy*, University of Rochester Press, p. 230.

6. Szreter, S. (2007) *Health and Wealth: Studies in History and Policy*, University of Rochester Press.

7. McKeown, T. (1976) *Modern Population*, Edward Arnold, p. 102.

8. Szreter, S. (2007) *Health and Wealth: Studies in History and Policy*, University of Rochester Press.

9. Ibid., p. 105.

10. Ibid., p. 32.

11. See for example Engels, F. (1973) *The Conditions of the Working Class*, Lawrence Wishart; see also, Cook, G.C., Thomas Southwood Smith FRCP (1788–1861): Leading exponent of diseases of poverty, and pioneer of sanitary reform in the mid-nineteenth century, *Journal of Medical Biography*, 10:4, pp. 194–205 (2002).

12. Szreter, S. (2007) *Health and Wealth: Studies in History and Policy*, University of Rochester Press, p. 120.

13. Wohl, A. (1983) *Endangered Lives: Public Health in Victorian Britain*, Cambridge University Press.

14. Szreter, S. (2007) *Health and Wealth: Studies in History and Policy*, University of Rochester Press, p. 121.

15. Taylor-Gooby, P. and Dale, J. (1981) *Social Theory and Social Welfare*, Edward Arnold.

16. Butterworth, E. and Holman, R. (1975) *Social Welfare in Modern Britain*, Fontana, p. 57–8.
17. Taylor-Gooby, P. and Dale, J. (1981) *Social Theory and Social Welfare*, Edward Arnold, pp. 156.
18. Hay, J. (1975) *The Origins of the Liberal Welfare Reforms 1906–1914*, Macmillan, p. 6.
19. Ibid., p. 6.
20. See for example Saville, J. (1987) *1848: The British State and the Chartist Movement*, Cambridge University Press; Thompson, D. (1984) *The Chartists*, Wildwood House.
21. Stearns, P. (1974) *The Revolutions of 1848*, Weidenfeld and Nicolson.
22. Marx, K. (1937) *The Eighteenth Brumaire of Louis Bonaparte*, Progress Publishers, chapter 7, www.marxists.org/archive/marx/works/1852/18th-brumaire/.
23. Flick, C. (1978) *The Birmingham Political Union and the Movements for Reform in Britain, 1830–1839*, Archon Books, p. 127.
24. Ibid., pp. 128–9.
25. Saville, J. (1987) *1848: The British State and the Chartist Movement*, Cambridge University Press, p. 145.
26. Flick, C. (1978) *The Birmingham Political Union and the Movements for Reform in Britain, 1830–1839*, Archon Books, p. 127.
27. Saville, J. (1987) *1848: The British State and the Chartist Movement*, Cambridge University Press, pp. 130–99; Goodway, D. (1982) *London Chartism 1838–1848*, Cambridge University Press.
28. For analysis of the role of trade union officials, see Cliff, T. and Gluckstein, D. (1986) *Marxism and Trade Union Struggle: The General Strike of 1926*, Bookmarks.
29. Hyman, R. (1975) *Industrial Relations: A Marxist Introduction*, Macmillan.
30. Ibid., p. 130.
31. Flick, C. (1978) *The Birmingham Political Union and the Movements for Reform in Britain, 1830–1839*, Archon Books, p. 131.
32. Bottomore, T. (1991) *A Dictionary of Marxist Thought*, Blackwell, cited in Stearns, P. (1974) *The Revolutions of 1848*, Weidenfeld and Nicolson, p. 226.
33. Canguilhem, G. (1989) *The Normal and the Pathological*, Zone Books.

Chapter 9

1. See, for example, Mikkonen, J., Social determinants of health and health inequalities, Government of Canada, www.canada.ca/en/public-health/services/health-promotion/population-health/what-determines-health.html.

2. WHO, Commission on Social Determinants of Health (2008) *Closing the Gap in a Generation: Health Equity Through Action on the Social Determinants of Health*, World Health Organization.

3. Ibid., p. 50.

4. Lewis, J., From Sure Start to children's centres: An analysis of policy change in English early years programmes, *Journal of Social Policy*, 40:1, pp. 71–88 (January 2011).

5. WHO, Commission on Social Determinants of Health (2008) *Closing the Gap in a Generation: Health Equity Through Action on the Social Determinants of Health*, World Health Organization.

6. Grantham-McGregor, S., et al., Developmental potential in the first 5 years for children in developing countries, *Lancet*, 369:9555, pp. 60–706 (January 2007).

7. WHO, Ten facts on obesity (October 2017) www.who.int/features/factfiles/obesity/en/.

8. Chakrabortty, A., What the great degree rip-off means for graduates: Low pay and high debt, *The Guardian* (19 April 2016), www.theguardian.com/commentisfree/2016/apr/19/degree-graduates-low-pay-high-debt-students.

9. Titmuss, R., Abel-Smith, B. and Titmuss, K. (eds) (1974) *Social Policy: An Introduction*, Pantheon Press, p. 107.

10. Waitzkin, H. (ed.) (2018) *Health Care Under the Knife: Moving Beyond Capitalism for Our Health*, Monthly Review Press, p. 107.

11. Marmot, M. and Wilkinson, R. (2006) *Social Determinants of Health* (2nd edition), Oxford University Press.

12. WHO, Commission on Social Determinants of Health (2008) *Closing the Gap in a Generation: Health Equity Through Action on the Social Determinants of Health*, World Health Organization.

13. Ibid.

14. Malthus, T.R. (2016) *Definitions in Political Economy*, Bocast, A.K. (ed.), Berkeley Bridge Press.

15. Ibid.

16. Meek, R. (1953) *Marx and Engels on the Population Bomb*, Ramparts Press.

17. Ibid., p. 76.

18. Ibid., pp. 76-7.

19. Maxwell , S. and Fernando, A., Cash crops in developing countries: The issues, the facts, the policies, *World Development*, 17:11, pp. 1677–708 (1989).

20. Holt-Gimenez, E. and Patel, R. (2009) *Food Rebellions: Crisis and the Hunger for Justice*, Pambazuka Press, p. 32.

21. Bello, W. (2009) *The Food Wars*, Verso, p. 68.

22. Mureithi, L., Coffee in Kenya: Some challenges for decent work, Sectoral Activities Programme Working Paper, International Labour Office, Geneva (2008).

23. See, for example, Wakefield, J., Apple Samsung and Sony face child labour claims, *BBC News* (19 January 2016), www.bbc.co.uk/news/technology-35311456.
24. Waitzkin, H. (ed.) (2018) *Health Care Under the Knife: Moving Beyond Capitalism for Our Health*, Monthly Review Press.
25. Ibid., p. 163.
26. Ibid., p. 164.
27. Ibid., p. 165.
28. Ibid., p. 167.
29. Ibid., p. 169.
30. Ibid., p. 169.
31. WHO, Commission on Social Determinants of Health (2008) *Closing the Gap in a Generation: Health Equity Through Action on the Social Determinants of Health*, World Health Organization.
32. Peoples Health Movement (2017) *Global Health Watch: An Alternative World Health Report*, Zed Books, pp. 278–97.
33. Ibid., p. 279.
34. Ibid., pp. 278–80.
35. Navaro, V. (ed.) (1979) *Imperialism Health and Medicine*, Baywood Publishing, p. 186.

Chapter 10

1. The Guillebaud Report, Report of the Committee of Enquiry into the cost of the National Health Service, Presented to Parliament by the Minister of Health and the Secretary of State for Scotland by Command of Her Majesty, January 1956, Cmd. 9663.
2. Webb, S. (2015) *The State and the Doctor*, Longmans.
3. Ibid., p. 211.
4. Holton, B. (1976) *British Syndicalism 1900–1914: Myths and Realities*, Pluto Press, pp. 73–5.
5. Pelling, H. (1967) *A History of British Trade Unions*, Palgrave, p. 261.
6. Holton, B. (1976) *British Syndicalism 1900–1914: Myths and Realities*, Pluto Press, 1976, p. 73.
7. Crowther, M. (1999) From workhouse to NHS hospital in Britain, 1929–1948, in Hillam, C. and Bon, J. (eds), *The Poor Law and After: Workhouse Hospitals and Public Welfare*, Liverpool Medical History Society, pp. 38–49.
8. Ibid., p. 105.
9. Stewart, J. (1999) *The Battle for Health: A Political History of the Socialist Medical Association 1930–51*, Ashgate, p. 1.
10. Navarro, V. (1978) *Class Struggle, the State and Medicine: An Historical and Contemporary Analysis of the Medical Sector in Great Britain*, Martin Robertson.

11. SHA (1934) *Labour Party Manifesto*, Socialist Health Association, www.sochealth.co.uk/socialism/labour-health-policy/.

12. Thane, P. (1996) *The Foundations of the Welfare State* (2nd edition), Longman.

13. Stark Murray, D. (1942) *Health for All*, Gollanz, p. 1.

14. Ibid., p. 65.

15. Earwicker, R. (1982) The labour movement and the creation of the National Health Service 1906–1948, unpublished PhD Thesis, University of Birmingham.

16. Abel-Smith, B. and Pinker, R. (1964) *The Hospitals, 1800–1948: A Study in Social Administration in England and Wales*, Harvard University Press, p. 424.

17. Earwicker, R. (1982) The labour movement and the creation of the National Health Service 1906–1948, unpublished PhD Thesis, University of Birmingham.

18. Pelling, H. (1967) *A History of British Trade Unions*, Palgrave, p. 83.

19. TUC History online, The labour movement and World War Two, www.unionhistory.info/timeline/1939_1945.php.

20. Clegg, H. (1994) *A History of British Trade Unions Since 1889, Volume III: 1934–1951*, Clarendon Press, pp. 169–72.

21. Dropkin, G., Strikes during wartime, labournet.net (29 May 2003), www.labournet.net/ukunion/0305/wartime1.html.

22. Clegg, H. (1994) *A History of British Trade Unions Since 1889, Volume III: 1934–1951*, Clarendon Press, p. 120.

23. Ibid., p. 156.

24. *The Economist*, His master's voice? (November 2000), www.economist.com/britain/2000/11/02/his-masters-voice.

25. Earwicker, R. (1982) The labour movement and the creation of the National Health Service 1906–1948, unpublished PhD Thesis, University of Birmingham.

26. Stewart, J. (1999) The Battle for Health: A Political History of the Socialist Medical Association 1930–51, Ashgate, pp. 168–70.

27. Bevan and the NHS, 1945–1948, The Development of the London Hospital System, 1823–2015, www.nhshistory.net/bevan.htm.

28. Rivett, G., Nye and the NHS, www.nyebevan.org.uk/nye-and-the-nhs/.

29. Rivett, G., The Development of the London Hospital System, 1823–2015: Bevan and the NHS, 1945–1948, www.nhshistory.net/bevan.htm.

30. Rivett, G., Nye and the NHS, www.nyebevan.org.uk/nye-and-the-nhs/.

31. Marx, K. (1937) *The Eighteenth Brumaire of Louis Bonaparte*, Progress Publishers, chapter 7, www.marxists.org/archive/marx/works/1852/18th-brumaire/.

32. Gale, A., 'I stuffed their mouths with gold': How hospitals destroyed the private practice of internal medicine, *Missouri Medicine*, 114:1, pp. 13–15 (January 2017).

33. Stewart, J. (1999) *The Battle for Health: A Political History of the Socialist Medical Association 1930–51*, Ashgate, p. 183.

34. Luxemburg, R., Reform or revolution, in Dick Howard (ed.) (1971) *Selected Political Writings of Rosa Luxemburg*, Monthly Review Press.

Index

AEU 69, 70, 126
Aging populations 13, 62, 64, 66, 68, 70–74, 76, 78, 96
Air pollution 143, 144
Alienation 87, 134
Appointed Day 119, 122, 129
Asthma 41, 42
Austerity 44, 58, 64, 70, 74, 133
Average life expectancy 29, 42, 60

Baby Boom 63, 64, 149
Beirne (P) 68, 149
Bevan (A) 119, 129–131, 134, 158
Bill and Melinda Gates Foundation (BMGF) 6, 13, 115, 116
Biomedical 1, 4, 5, 38, 40, 45, 75, 129
Black Report 9, 137
BMA 8, 122, 125, 128, 129
BMJ 11, 24, 137, 140, 141
Brayne (C) 76, 77, 151
British Social Attitudes 16, 119
Bronchitis 42, 99
Bukharin (N) 37–38, 92, 143, 153

Call centres 49, 146
Callahan (D) 71, 150
Cancer 23, 42, 45, 48, 51, 55, 58, 86
Canguilhem (G) 4, 5, 41, 107, 136, 145
Cardiovascular disease 43, 45, 58
Cash crops 113, 114, 116, 156
Centralisation 26, 34, 35, 38
Chadwick (E) 100, 106
Chamberlain (J) 106, 107
Chartism 102–106, 155
Child labour 51, 105, 108, 113, 115, 147, 157

Clinical Commissioning Group (CCG) 18, 19, 138, 150
Closing the Gap in a Generation (WHO) 7, 39, 108, 109, 110, 111, 116, 117, 137, 143, 156, 157
Coburn (D) 57–60, 134, 148
Commodification 13, 14, 19, 27
Corporate Europe Observatory 17, 137, 138

Dementia 45, 65, 76–78, 151
Demographic transition theory 96, 154
Dependency ratios 71, 72, 150
Diabetes 33, 45, 46, 58, 77, 86
Diet (see Chpt 4)
Dorling (D) 2, 8, 9, 10, 53, 65, 134, 137, 149

Emergency medical service (EMS) (see Chpt 10)
Engels (F) 44, 112, 113, 144, 154, 156
English Revolution 89, 91, 94
Eugenics 110, 111
Exploitation 17, 35–36, 102, 105, 106, 112, 114, 134, 135

Fabians 101, 128
Factory Acts 105
Fertility rates 109, 110, 111, 113, 114, 116, 118
Financial Times 21, 23, 138, 139
Food adulteration 46
Food crime unit 46, 145
Forbes 33, 139, 141, 142
Foucault (M) (see Chpt 7)
Free school milk 67
French Revolution (see Chpt 7)

General Practitioners (GPs) 19, 86, 122, 123
Giddens (A) 55, 136, 147
Goldfinger (E) 68, 149
Gould (S-J) 56, 57, 147

Health and Safety Executive 50, 52, 105, 146
Health bubble 37
Health paradigm 11, 37, 38, 90, 96, 133
Hippocrates 89–90
Homelessness 42–43, 68, 144
Housing (see Chpt 4)
Hypertension 45, 58, 77

Ideology 17, 83, 103, 107, 133, 149
Illich (I) 85–86, 152
Inequality Thesis (see Chpt 5)
International Labour Organisation (ILO) 51, 52, 109, 147, 156
Italy 43, 57, 60, 61, 73, 91, 102

Joseph Rowntree Foundation 74
Junior doctors 87, 153
Junk food 45, 46, 145

Kings Fund 16, 17, 137
Kuhn (T) 11, 18, 80, 82, 88, 93, 94, 138, 153, 154

Labisch (A) (see Chpt 7)
Labour Party 67, 91, 118, 122–125, 127, 128, 131, 132, 158
Lancet 42, 137, 147, 154, 156
LangBuisson 21, 24, 139, 140
Laski (H) 91, 123, 153
Learning disabilities 21, 25, 26, 120, 139, 140
Lower and Middle Income Countries (LMIC) 2, 44, 65, 108, 109, 113, 118

Malthus (T) 75, 111–112, 156

Manchester School 84
Marmot (M) 7–9, 10, 40, 53, 54, 56, 64, 65, 70, 111, 134, 137, 147, 149, 156
Marx (K) 35, 36, 87, 104, 105, 112, 131, 155, 156, 158
McKeown Thesis 96, 97, 154
Medicaid 30–33, 141
Medical gaze 80, 83, 86, 87, 151
Medical industrial complex 140, 142
Medicare 30, 31, 32, 141
Mental health 5, 7, 18, 42–44, 86, 120, 144, 145, 146
Mergers and acquisitions 21, 33, 54
Middling Sort 94
Ministry of Food 65, 66
Minority Report 120

National Food Survey 66
Neoliberalism 12–13, 14, 19, 44, 58, 59, 133, 137
Newsholme (A) 91, 92, 153
NHS (see Chpts 2 & 10)
Nordic Countries 59

Obamacare 30, 32, 141
Obesity 7, 34, 45, 46, 58, 77, 110, 156
Observationes Medicae 89–90
OECD 29, 30, 60, 74, 75
Office for National Statistics 64, 152
Older people (see Chpt 6)
Ottawa Charter for Health Promotion 3–6, 136
Overpopulation 70, 111, 118
Oxfordshire 14, 21, 138

PAC hospitals 121
Panel Doctors 120
Paradigm shift 11, 82, 88, 95, 135
Pensioner poverty 74, 151
Pensions Myth 72, 76, 150, 151
Philanthrocapitalism 6, 13, 22, 115, 118, 133
Pickett (K) 2, 7, 9, 10, 53, 57, 58, 134, 136, 137, 147, 148

Poor Law 103, 104, 120–122, 157

Population growth 96–101, 112

Porter (R) 89, 97, 151, 153, 154

Pre-fabs 67

Public-Private-Partnership (PPP) 5, 6, 13, 16, 115, 116, 117

Reserve army of labour 112, 113

Royal College of Physicians 89, 131

Russian Revolution 11, 37, 91, 93, 94, 153

Sans Culottes 94

Semashko (N) 92, 93, 153

Smith (A) 36, 100, 112, 143

Social cohesion theory 56, 58, 60, 61, 148

Social construction of health 84, 152

Social determinants of health (see Chpt 4)

Social impact investment 22, 139

Socialist Medical Association 122, 157, 158, 159

Standing committee on nutrition 110

Suicide 42, 55, 67, 86, 114, 152, 153

Sure Start 108, 109, 156

Surplus population 112

Sydenham (T) 88–90, 153

Szreter (S) 97–100, 106, 154

Tawney (RH) 94, 153

Taylor-Goody (P) 102

Technology 14, 24, 34, 37, 49, 83, 115, 133, 140, 157

Toxic waste 41

Tuberculosis 43, 44, 45, 117, 145

Universal credit 59–60

Valeant Pharmacy 33

Voodoo demography 63, 71, 72

Webb (S & B) 101, 120, 122, 157

Weber (M) 55, 147

Whitehall Studies 7, 54–55, 56, 57, 136, 147

Wilkinson (E) 67

Wilkinson (R) 7, 10, 52–53, 57, 58, 111, 134, 136, 137, 148, 156

World Bank 44, 109, 117, 118, 142

World Health Organisation (WHO) (see Chpt 9)

World War I 63, 94, 120

World War II 1, 12, 41, 42, 45, 63, 64, 65, 66, 69, 78, 79, 91, 110, 111, 120

Zombie business 23, 139